MW01172391

The ultimate
Anti-Inflammatory Cookbook For
Diabetes

A 60-Day Ultimate Anti-Inflammatory Recipe Guide to Healthy Eating and Diabetes Management (Include 30 days meal Plan)

Tony Harrell

1

About the author

Tony Harrell was born in North Texas in 1988. She is a chef and nutritionist from the USA. She graduated from the College of Nutrition and Food Science at the University of North Carolina. Then she worked under a health specialist for 2 years. This book is part of her passion of writing and personal experiences.

Table of Contentes

Introduction

Although living with diabetes might be difficult, it does not imply that you have to give up taste and satisfaction when it comes to the food you eat due to the condition. The significance of maintaining a healthy and balanced diet in the management of diabetes is something that I have seen directly as a healthcare practitioner who has dealt with a large number of diabetic patients over the course of my career. Finding breakfast alternatives that are not only nutritional and healthy but also tasty and enjoyable is one of the most difficult issues that many individuals who have diabetes face. This is the reason why I was so excited when I was contacted with the concept of writing a cookbook that would be centered particularly on breakfast foods that are suitable for diabetics.

This book has a broad range of breakfast ideas that are designed to cater to a variety of preferences and tastes throughout the day. This book offers everything you could possibly need, whether you are searching for breakfasts that are simple and quick to prepare on busy weekdays, breakfasts that are low in carbohydrates to assist in managing your blood sugar levels, breakfasts that are rich in protein to keep you feeling full and content, or three international meals to add some variation to your morning routine. This cookbook, however, is not just comprised of recipes. In the first chapter, you will discover an introduction to diabetes and an explanation of how it impacts breakfast, as well as some suggestions for preparing a meal that is nutritionally sound. You will also gain knowledge on typical breakfast blunders that you should avoid making, such as missing breakfast entirely or depending on items that are high in sugar for breakfast. For your convenience, the appendix contains example meal plans and recipes that will assist you in putting the recipes included in this book into action. With careful consideration, these meal plans have been crafted to provide a diet that is both well-balanced and diverse, while also taking into account the various calorie and carbohydrate requirements of individuals. I really hope that this cookbook will motivate you to be creative in the kitchen and enjoy some wonderful breakfasts that are suitable for people with diabetes. As long as you have the appropriate components and a little bit of knowledge, you can get your day off to a good start and feel your very best.

My experience as someone who lives with and treats people who have diabetes has given me an understanding of how stressful it can be to find breakfast alternatives that are not only tasty but also gratifying and suitable for diabetics. This cookbook was written with the intention of assisting those who suffer from diabetes in savoring delectable meals that are not only nutritious but also filled with taste. The recipes included in this book have been meticulously designed to make sure that they contain an appropriate proportion of carbs, protein, and healthy fats, in addition to being bursting with flavor and texture. There is something for everyone in this cookbook, from breakfasts that are quick and simple to prepare for hectic mornings to eleven alternatives for slow cookers that are perfect for laid-back weekends. This cookbook, however, is not just comprised of recipes. Additionally, it provides useful information on diabetes and breakfast, such as the significance of consuming a well-balanced meal and the typical errors that should be avoided while eating breakfast. Through the use of this knowledge, readers will be able to make educated judgments on the breakfast options they choose, positioning themselves for success throughout the day. In the first chapter, you will discover an introduction to diabetes and an explanation of how it impacts breakfast, as well as some suggestions for preparing a meal that is nutritionally sound. You will also gain knowledge on typical breakfast blunders that you should avoid making, such as missing breakfast entirely or depending on items that are high in sugar for breakfast. The purpose of this chapter is to provide readers with the knowledge necessary to comprehend the significance of a nutritious breakfast and to learn how to make decisions that will be beneficial to their health and well-being.

Chapter 1

Inflammation

Inflammation is the body's formal acknowledgment to shield itself from damage. There are two types- Acute plus Chronic. You're more familiar; including some distinctive style that happens while you bump you're Knee or cutting your Finger. Your immune system confers soldiers of White Blood Cells to enclose and preserve the area, making prominent Redness and Swelling.

This method operates the same if you possess an infection such as Flu or Pneumonia. Hence, Ignition is essential. Without it, Injuries can become severe-plus plain Infections can be lethal.

Chronic Inflammation

Chronic Inflammation can further transpire response through another undesired object in the body, before-mentioned while Toxins of Cigarette Smoke or excess Fatty Cells (Particularly Belly Fat). In the Arteries; Inflammation improves Trigger Atherosclerosis, the quantity of Fatty Plaque rich in Cholesterol.

Your body notices this Plaque as unusual and unfamiliar, So it attempts to obstruct the Plaque so that this Blood does not move. But if that Wall Breaks, this plate can separate. These contents later combine with the Blood to create a Clot that Blocks Blood Flow. These clots form most utmost Heart Attacks and Strokes.

Symptoms of Chronic Inflammation

The most noticeable sign connected with Inflammation is Joint Pain, though several different methods manifest Inflammation in the body. If persistent digestive difficulties are linked to Stomach pain, Bloating, and irritating bowels, it occurs in the Intestines. Skin difficulties like Eczema and Psoriasis are different processes. Inflammation exposes itself further overtly. Some sorts of Inflammation are complex and can perform unrecognized. For Example, if you are Overweight or Obese, your body will undergo Inflammation because fat cells transmit Chemical Messages that enhance Inflammation. Having High Cholesterol or High Blood Sugar also begins the Inflammatory process in the body. It's the alliance regarding High Cholesterol with Inflammation that significantly enhances the chance of heart disease.

Diet Affect Inflammation

Numerous particular components in a Gluten-free Diet linked with an Anti-inflammatory diet. Note, everyone acknowledges food differently. This consolidation of some or a total of specific systems remains one of them.

Diet can assist with accurate and Long-term health advantages. Reducing Gluten from this Diet [particularly in very processed from White Flour also Sugar] will promote wellness.

Moreover, eliminate Highly Processed Meat [several containing Gluten as an Additive] performs this method activity.These results might be extra progressive in unusual forms if questioned Doctor whence due to Chronic Illness.

The difference in an Anti-inflammatory or Gluten-free Diet may arise to resolve this thorny way to healthier Health. An Anti-inflammatory Diet can create numerous health interests.

Anti-inflammatory Diet

The Anti-Inflammatory diet can manage signs by diminishing the conclusions of Inflammation. This diet limits few foods while promoting and suggests consuming at a particular moment of the Day to affect Inflammation.

An Anti-Inflammatory diet concentrates on consuming Plant Foods plus Fish, rich in good Fats and Phytonutrient while maintaining Blood Sugar. In that fact, this diet intends to change the Control Mechanisms that regulate this Inflammatory method.

The Anti-Inflammatory Diet is based on a Mediterranean-Style consumption method involving many Vegetables; Fruits; Legumes; Nuts; Seeds; Healthy oils; and Fish. It is further designated the Pescatarian Diet because Fish is the primary origin of Animal Protein, and the most effective form of diet consists of Plant Foods.

An essential phase of an Anti-Inflammatory Diet is a Low-Glycemic Diet, which indicates that your Blood Sugar does not stand and decline throughout that Day.

Polished Grains and Sugar are regularly toward some standard American Diet and moderate in Fiber. That mixture results in Excess Sugar in the Blood. Our bodies can become indifferent to the Insulin Signal that serves us to transport Glucose to our Fuel Cells throughout that occurs over a lengthy period. For this reason, too much Glucose will drift wherever it does not, uttering the alerts that trigger this Inflammatory Response.

There are various causes that kind above of consumption retains Inflammation at bay, though the several influential Superstar above a Pescatarian Diet is:

OMEGA-3 fatty acid:

Located primarily inside Shellfish and in shorter Walnuts; Flax; and some Green Leafy Vegetables Similar Kale. Omega-3 Fatty Acids are a collection of Unsaturated Fats which defend the body from Inflammation in several methods.

Fiber:

Fiber is located in Plant Foods like Fruits; Vegetables; Whole grains, and Nuts. Fiber is an unchangeable portion of certain foods and is essential for healthful Digestion, Blood Sugar, and Cholesterol control. A high-fiber diet and below levels of Inflammatory labels in the Blood.

Carotenoids:

Located in Carrots; Garnet Root; Pumpkin, and Cantaloupe, Beta-carotene and other carotenoids seem risky at Inflammatory Arthritis.

Vitamin K:

Located in Leafy Green Vegetables such as Swiss Kale and Cardamom; Brussels Sprouts; Broccoli; Cabbage, and Seafood. Vitamin K is a vital nutrient that helps improve Inflammatory methods in this body. That also signifies a potent Antioxidant through diminishing Oxidative Stress that can lead to Inflammation.

Magnesium:

Located in Leafy Green Vegetables; Nuts; Seeds; Legumes; and Whole Grains. Magnesium is amongst the most leading on the listing of Minerals that resemble to defend against Inflammation.

Anti-Inflammatory Diet Effective or Not?

We each hold a different Immune System that reacts separately to several situations.

The consequences per Nutritional Protocol will diversify from Person to Person. Other constituents include Adherence to the diet and involvement definite difference. Linked with the complexity of the Inflammatory Method, this describes why numerous People with Inflammatory states favor a Multidisciplinary method to assist them in managing their situation. An Anti-Inflammatory diet can be an element of this method, except it may not relieve Inflammation on its individual. It maintained the testimony holds that an Anti-Inflammatory diet can alleviate signs or assist as a worthy accessory to pharmaceutical or Physical interferences, producing daily alerts further controllable.

Beneficial Condition of Anti-Inflammatory Diet

It is well established that inflammation is thought to be the root cause of several long-term illnesses. Lupus and rheumatoid arthritis are examples of autoimmune disorders; cancer, heart disease, diabetes, gastrointestinal problems, depression, and dementia are among them.Some inflammatory conditions, such as obesity and overweight, might have their own risk factors influenced by lifestyle and diet. Especially, endanger yourself greatly. When there is an overabundance of inflammatory messengers, the result is excessive adipose tissue, and this silent inflammatory condition is known as obesity. Because it causes pain, it is said to be silent.

Furthermore, this may lead to type 2 diabetes, metabolic syndrome, and systemic inflammation in the long run.There is a genetic link to several inflammatory conditions. Skin disorders like eczema and psoriasis are part of the atopic conditions category, which also includes asthma and allergies.

Chapter 2

Nutrition and Diabetes

Diabetes is a metabolic disease that is characterized by problems controlling blood glucose levels. The inability of the pancreas to generate enough insulin is the hallmark of type 1 diabetes, whereas the body's incapacity to use the insulin that is produced appropriately is the hallmark of type 2 diabetes. Diabetes might occur as a result of any of these situations. In the United States, diabetes affects around 29 million people, or over 9.3% of the population. That being said, one in four people with diabetes is not aware that they have the illness. Ninety-five percent of those with a diabetes diagnosis have type 2 diabetes, whereas five percent have type 1 diabetes. Overweight or obese people make up a significant part of those with type 2 diabetes diagnoses. When a person is overweight or obese, the body finds it more challenging to use the insulin the pancreas produces to transfer sugar into the body's cells. Reduced weight may help people with type 2 diabetes because it promotes fat cell loss, which can improve the body's ability to produce and use insulin more effectively. Diabetes not only significantly affects a person's health, but it also significantly affects the whole health care system. A person diagnosed with diabetes has a fifty percent higher risk of dying throughout their adult lifetime. Individuals with diabetes are more likely to have a number of unfavorable health consequences, such as blindness, renal failure, heart disease, stroke, amputation of the toes, feet, or legs, and improper kidney function.

Diabetes management using medical nutrition therapy

When it comes to managing diabetes mellitus, medical nutrition therapy (MNT) is often regarded as the most crucial component (Kodama et al., 2009). Inadequate regulation of blood pressure, cholesterol, and glucose levels may lead to serious complications, which is why MNT is so important for preventing and controlling diabetes. For each phase of diabetes prevention, MNT is crucial, as stated in the Nutrition Recommendations and Interventions for Diabetes by ADA.

1.   Primary prevention: preventing diabetes in obese and pre-diabetic persons by using MNT and public health interventions;
2.   Secondary prevention: using MNT for type 1, type 2, and gestational diabetes metabolic management to avoid complications;
3.   Tertiary prevention: using MNT to postpone and control in order to avoid morbidity and death.

TheADA and the AND both recommend that people with prediabetes, type 1 and type 2 diabetes, as well as populations affected by metabolic and glycemic disruption, receive MNT from a registered dietitian nutritionist (RD/RDN) (AND, 2011; ADA, 2015). It is recommended that the team member responsible for providing nutrition care be a registered dietitian nutritionist (RDN) with expertise in MNT; however, other team members and practitioners must also be knowledgeable about MNT for diabetes.

Risk Factors for Diabetes

Type 1 diabetes is a genetic condition that is often diagnosed in younger individuals, such as children and young adults. People with type 1 diabetes need frequent insulin injections to help move sugar from meals into their bodies' cells since they are unable to produce insulin on their own. Type 1 diabetes is not entirely understood to be caused by a single factor; nonetheless, there is a slight chance that an individual may get the disease if family members already have it. The International Diabetes Federation (2014) states that exposure to viruses and some environmental factors are associated with the development of type 1 diabetes. 38 - Illnesses and Medical Care One of the main characteristics of type 2 diabetes is insulin resistance, which is the body's incapacity to use insulin as needed. The following are some risk factors for type 2 diabetes:

• Being overweight and/or physically sedentary;

• A family history of diabetes is a risk factor.

• If you had diabetes while you were pregnant or if you had a history of inadequate nutrition during pregnancy

• Compared to other groups of individuals, Asian Americans, African Americans, Mexican Americans, American Indians, Native Hawaiians, and residents of Pacific Islands are more likely to acquire diabetes. by smoking;

• An aging populace

• An increased pulse rate as stated by the IDF (2014)

The Importance of Diet

With the adoption of a diet that is both healthy and balanced, it is possible to start eliminating many of the issues that are related with waste buildup in the body. Moreover, it supplies the body with sufficient nutrients that are necessary for maintaining a proper equilibrium. The digestive system is responsible for incorporating food into the body, converting it into usable energy via the process of nutrient absorption, and eliminating waste products that cannot be used in an effective manner. If the food we consume is of a better quality, then we will acquire a greater quantity of nutrients and energy from it.

Reducing the Impact of the Overload of Toxic Substances

On a daily basis, we are exposed to environmental pollutants as well as dietary byproducts that have accumulated as a result of our diet. In the process of consuming non-useful chemicals that are found in meals, such as hormones, pesticides, antibiotic residues, and other compounds, our bodies are required to exert additional effort in order to digest these alien substances. This is in addition to the fact that they are acquiring nutrients from such foods. Because they are in charge of the metabolism of harmful chemicals, the liver and kidneys are required to work hard in order to break down toxins that come from our surroundings, the food we eat, and the metabolic processes that we go through. The efficiency with which the human body accomplishes metabolic processes is not one hundred percent. Typically, it results in the production of wastes and endogenous toxins, both of which need to be processed and eliminated from the body. The "terrain" of a person is determined by the efficiency with which their body eliminates these accumulated wastes. Terrain refers to the sensitivity of the body to illness attributable to the biochemical and energetic environment in which it operates. The implication of this is that various people have distinct terrains or environments. In addition to toxins found in the environment and certain foods, pharmaceutical medications are another type of toxins that come from the outside. The liver and kidneys are the primary organs responsible for catabolizing, or breaking down, these poisons and excreting them from the body thereafter. Lastly, in addition to the responsibility of metabolizing wastes and poisons, the body must also be able to digest and break down allergens that are inhaled via the air or ingested through food. Does the fact that we are collecting more poisons cause our systems to get overloaded make any sense? Does it also make sense that limiting the amount of toxins we consume may improve the efficiency with which we remove the ones that are still present?

The following is an example that can assist you in understanding the ability of the body to deal with stress, toxins, allergies, and metabolic wastes, as well as how these factors may be related to your diet. Imagine that you have a cup that can accommodate eight ounces of drinking liquid. There is a possibility that you are consuming allergens and toxins via this cup. In the event that you fill the cup with six ounces of food allergens, you will only be able to take in two more ounces before the cup overflows and you are no longer able to cope with the potentially harmful substances. In the event that you are then subjected to environmental contaminants, pollens during the springtime, and pharmaceutical medicines, your cup will not be able to manage all of the assaults that are being directed against your system. Your cup may overflow, causing you to suffer a variety of symptoms, including discomfort, a runny nose, postnasal drip, cough, rash, exhaustion, and many more (which will be covered further on in the part which is dedicated to food allergies). The flip side of the coin is that if you get rid of the six ounces of food allergies, you will have a greater capacity to take in and digest allergens and poisons that you cannot avoid. Patients who suffer from severe allergies to grass and pollen, for instance, are unable to exclude all grass and pollen from their life. However, they may reduce their food allergies in order to enable their bodies to more effectively absorb grass and pollen.

Adhere to a healthy diet when dealing with type 2 diabetes

One of the most important factors defining our overall health, energy, and well-being is what we eat. Ingesting a large quantity of food causes a cascade of reactions that culminate in the absorption of glucose into the bloodstream. The pancreas produces insulin, which humans rely on to regulate blood glucose levels. Keeping glucose levels from being dangerously high or low is a top priority. You will know that your pancreas isn't making enough insulin or that the insulin it does make isn't working properly if you have type 2 diabetes. Diabetes is linked to both of these outcomes. A complete lack of insulin production is an indicator of type 1 diabetes.

The importance of what you eat is paramount for those with type 2 diabetes. All people should strive to eat healthily, but those with diabetes should do so with more vigor. With the right food choices, you may lessen your chances of developing diabetes-related complications and maybe even aid in the control of your illness. Following a regimen similar to ours, which includes carrot-ginger soup and summer pudding, helped individuals with type 2 diabetes lower their blood glucose levels by 25% on average, according to one study. This is what the researchers found. Rather than focusing on whether or not your supper was delicious, try to eat a variety of things throughout the day. In the realm of cuisine, one can't definitively claim victory. Despite the frequent discussion of good and terrible dishes, there is no such thing as a better or worse meal.

Consume a diet rich in fresh produce

Adding more veggies to your diet is an easy way to improve your nutrition. At each meal, aim to have half of your plate filled with vegetables. However, you shouldn't think of them as only an accessory; instead, you should see them as a component that you can include in your favorite cuisines. Antioxidant vitamins, minerals, and phytochemicals abound in vegetables, and they're low in calories and high in fiber. Many of the complications associated with diabetes may be lessened if people with diabetes eat more vegetables. Eating fruit may help lower the risk of cardiovascular disease, several cancers, and gastrointestinal problems, according to some research. Fruit also contains several of the essential minerals and vitamins. Keep in mind that fruit contains natural carbohydrates that might impact your blood glucose level; hence, it's best to avoid eating a bunch of fruit at once. Fruit juice has a lot more sugar that is quickly released into the bloodstream compared to dried fruit, which is a concentrated source of these sugars; hence, it is better to eat whole, fresh fruit instead of fruit juice.

Satiating appetite

If you're attempting to lose weight by cutting down on food intake, you could find it challenging to keep from becoming hungry. A calorie-conscious diet that promotes satiety rather than hunger may help you avoid this problem. You will feel full, or satisfied, after eating, but how much food you eat determines how strong that feeling is. For those interested in the details, there is a technique called the satiety index that assesses meals based on their ability to satisfy hunger. There are several important factors to think about, but one of the most basic is the quantity of food you consume. Keep in mind that a relatively tiny quantity of cheese has a lot of calories, so if you nibble on it regularly, you should limit yourself to that amount. Picking this over fresh produce increases the likelihood that you will be dissatisfied. This is because eating a lot of fruits and veggies won't make you gain weight since they are low in calories. Here we see how different portions of meals with the same total calories stack up against one another. The healthy fruit and vegetable options on the right make it easy to eat more, so you won't be hungry until the next meal.

Cholesterol and diet

Can cholesterol levels be elevated by consuming foods rich in cholesterol?

Although this is true for 30% of the population, the vast majority of individuals do not experience a rise in cholesterol levels after consuming meals that are rich in cholesterol. About three-quarters of the cholesterol our bodies produce comes from the decomposition of meals. What we consume provides the remaining energy. Consuming extra cholesterol causes either a decrease in body production or its breakdown and excretion by the liver. Red meat, poultry, eggs, dairy products (including ice cream, butter, and cheese), and veal all include saturated animal fats. Choose low-fat dairy products, such as yogurt, milk, and cheese. Make an effort to eat less fat. According to the majority of research, eating fish may lessen your risk of heart disease and raise your levels of good cholesterol (HDL). The heart-healthy omega-3 fatty acids EPA and DHA (docosahexaenoic acid) are present in fish oil, and fish is low in saturated fat.

Consuming vegetables is highly advised. The natural constriction of your body's arteries, brought about by their abundance of antioxidants, breaks down harmful oxidized cholesterol and keeps it from blocking your arteries. It is believed that partially hydrogenated vegetable oils are harmful to the heart. Unsaturated vegetable oils, which are full of unstable molecules and might become rancid, should be avoided at all costs. The majority of vegetable oils include unsaturated fats. Canola and olive oils, which are both monounsaturated, are suggested. As a healthy fat, butter is also highly recommended. You must use olive oil moderately if you want to enjoy its deliciousness, nutritional density, and pleasant aroma.

What causes high cholesterol?

There are many risk factors for high cholesterol (hypercholesterolemia), including (but not in no particular order):

- Familial hypercholesterolemia (hereditary genetic disease)

- High sugar intake (significantly refined sugar)

- High intake of saturated fats

- Any intake of trans fats

- Low activity level, lack of exercise

- Hyperreactivity (i.e. your baseline cholesterol level is low, but any dietary intake raises it significantly)

- Intestinal flora (some bacteria can convert cholesterol into inert and indigestible substances)

- Stress, both physical and mental. moderate correlation*

Interestingly, here are some things that are NOT risk factors for high cholesterol:

- High cholesterol intake (unless you are hypersensitive) does not affect blood cholesterol levels (within certain limits, but expected).

- Smoking and drinking alcohol (oxidizes cholesterol, making it harmful and more likely to cause problems in the future, but levels stay the same)

- Sun exposure (vitamin D production does not affect cholesterol levels; the liver will produce more to keep it within normal limits)

These factors often occur together, so mixing them in studies is difficult. Therefore, it's better to maintain the optimum cholesterol level.

High Blood Pressure

Cardiovascular failure risk starts with hypertension. Hypertension builds the gamble of coronary illness, renal disappointment, strokes, and mortality. Hypertension is destructive. Hypertension, known as "the quiet executioner," has no side effects until it causes a deadly cardiovascular failure or stroke. Systolic and diastolic circulatory strain are two qualities. The U.S. Public Establishments of Wellbeing characterizes typical systolic strain as 120 mmHg or less and diastolic as 80 or less. 95% of hypertension is fundamental, meaning it isn't brought about by a growth or renal disease. Fundamental hypertension is delivered by atherosclerosis-solidified veins that increment fringe obstruction. Thoughtful sensory system movement is another variable. Long haul salt utilization causes this more troublesome condition. With its low-supplement, handled, high-glycemic-load dinners and creature items, the Miserable causes constant second rate endothelial brokenness. Horrible eating routines produce oxidative pressure, or far-reaching aggravation, because of free extremists.

Substitute Healthier Ingredients

Our body plays out an extraordinary number and assortment of capabilities all through a day, a considerable lot of which require quite certain supplements. Remembered for this rundown of capabilities is, obviously, the recuperating system. But since the overall population periodically has little information on what is required healthfully to reestablish and keep up with their bodies, their frameworks need key components, which should be added through external sources. Whether you're hoping to engage your body to recuperate, wanting to achieve a full illness inversion, or hoping to accomplish an ideal degree of progress, certain way of life changes — alongside meeting key dietary necessities — are required. Coming up next is a bunch of proposals, expected on a continuous premise, for anybody needing to accomplish health and keep an illness precaution way of life.

Quit Separating the Body

The initial step is to stop making any further lopsided characteristics inside your body while lessening any known givers for sickness. For instance, assuming you smoke, either quit smoking or incredibly decline your everyday sum. On the off chance that your eating routine is too high in acidic substances (which can cause irritation and make safe aggravations), most prominently espresso, liquor and sweet and jazzed refreshments, diminish your admission of these issue food sources. Stay away from boring food varieties, tissue protein, and sugar, and lower or kill your utilization of destructive, synthetic loaded food substances, including illuminated salt, synthetic compounds, handled meat items, pop, prepackaged food, white flour and white rice, synthetic sugars, and food with additives.

Treating and Preventing High Blood Pressure

Everybody ought to have their circulatory strain minded a standard premise. Assuming your circulatory strain is high, it is essential to look for exhortation and take on way of life changes that will assist with diminishing your pulse. For a great many people, the way of life changes framed in this part will be adequate to control pulse. For other people, typically those at stage 2 hypertension, such changes are inadequate and physician endorsed prescriptions are expected to control pulse. However, in any event, for those getting pharmacologic treatment, adjusting these solid way of life changes is in any case basic since they effectively upgrade the adequacy of prescriptions. At anything stage you find yourself, there are five key way of life changes that you can embrace to forestall or decrease your gamble of growing hypertension. These will be examined thusly in this part and extensively incorporate the accompanying: staying away from salt, taking on a sound eating regimen, keeping away from destructive substances, practicing consistently, and overseeing pressure.

Chapter 3

Breakfasts

1. Turkey Breakfast Sausage

Ingredients:

- Turkey chunks
- Rolled oats (20 g)
- Two tbsp of oat wheat
- Two tablespoons of buttered wheat cereal, such as Wheaten (about 18 grams) (around 18 g)
- Cooking pop, one teaspoon
- Cornstarch, a teaspoon's worth
- One-tenth of a tsp of vanilla extract
- ½ cup (355 grams) of nonfat milk
- 2 egg whites

Procedures:

- The components should be mixed together well.
- Cook in a hot frying pan, on a grill, or in a heated cooker at 325F on a greased baking sheet.

2. Breakfast in the Snow Casserole

Ingredients:

- 2 slices of bacon with reduced salt
- Shredded 3 potatoes
- Chopped onion, about half a cup (80 grams)
- Diced green bell pepper
- 4 eggs
- 30 grams (about a quarter cup) of low-fat Shredded Cheddar Cheese

Procedures:

- Turn on cooker to 350F.
- Cook the bacon in a weighty container.
- Take the bacon out and allow it to deplete on a platter fixed with paper towels.
- Heat the potatoes, onion, and green pepper until the potatoes are firm and the onions are delicate in a skillet.
- Throw in some bacon bits.

- Continue to put in a square baking dish that is 8 creeps in size and has been oiled.
- Add beaten eggs and serve.
- Spread some cheddar on top.
- Around 20 minutes in the stove ought to get the job done.

3.   Skillet for Breakfast

Originally, we would have this for breakfast on a Sunday in late summer. This dish helped me use up some of the excess peppers that I always have at that time of year from my garden.

Ingredients:

- 15 milliliters (1 tablespoon) olive oil a quarter of a cup (40 grams) of finely chopped onion
- Finely sliced red bell pepper (about 38 grams)
- Brown potatoes, thawed
- 3 beaten eggs

Procedures:

- Set up a major skillet with oil and intensity it over medium intensity. Red ringer peppers and onions ought to be cooked in olive oil until delicate.
- Hash browns ought to be added and cooked, blending occasionally, until they are delicate and beginning to brown.
- Mix the eggs to the veggies and stew for an extra 5 minutes, mixing occasionally, until the eggs have set.

As a portion:

- 13g- protein
- 10g-total fat
- 13g-carbohydrates
- 1g-fiber per serving;
- 195kj

4.   Vegetable Omelet

Either a morning meal or the centerpiece of supper.

Ingredients:

- 2 ounces (55 grams) sliced mushrooms;
- 1/4 cup (40 grams) chopped onion
- Olive oil, one tablespoon (around 15 ml)
- Diced green bell peppers, about a quarter cup (37 g)
- Toss up some zucchini and tomatoes for some veggie-packed flavor!
- 4 eggs

- Fat-free sour cream equivalent to 2 teaspoons (30 g)
- Just under 2 teaspoons (30 ml) of water
- Swiss cheese, shredded; 2 ounces (55 g)

Procedure:

- In an enormous container, warm the olive oil and sauté the mushrooms, onion, green ringer pepper, zucchini, and tomato until the vegetables are delicate.
- Eggs, harsh cream, and water might be sped into a light and vaporous hitter.
- Shower a skillet or omelet container with nonstick veggie splash and intensity it over medium intensity. Break eggs into a skillet.
- For an uncooked egg to stream underneath the cooked surface, lift the edges as it cooks.
- At the point when the eggs are practically finished, flip over the uncooked piece and top it with the cheddar and sautéed veggies.

5.   Omelet with cinnamon and apples

A tasty twist on the traditional breakfast food. Recipes for omelets stuffed with jelly or other sweet fillings used to be more common than they are now, but I recall when that used to be the case. Thanks to this one, I now believe they are worthwhile.

Ingredients:

- One tablespoon of unsalted butter, split
- One apple, thinly cut and peeled
- 1/4 of a teaspoon of ginger
- Brown sugar, one tablespoon's worth (15 g)
- 3 eggs
- Exactly 1 Tablespoon of Cream
- Sour cream, one tablespoon

Procedures:

- Set up an egg skillet by softening 2 tablespoons of spread in it. Mix in certain apples, flavors, and dim sugar.
- The vegetables ought to be sautéed till delicate.
- Place to the side. Cushy egg and cream will be whipped and left to the side. Clean the egg skillet.
- Add the excess egg combination to the dissolved margarine.
- Techniques like those utilized for making an omelet ought to be utilized.
- At the point when the eggs are cooked, flip them and spoon some harsh cream in the center.
- Top with the apple combination. Organize it collapsed on a dish.

As a portion:

- 11g-protein,
- 110mg-phosphorus,
- 73mg-calcium,
- 2mg-iron,
- 40mg-sodium,

6. Quiche with Spinach

This recipe is so adaptable that you can consume it at every time of the day.

Ingredients:

- Reduced-sodium bacon in 8 slices
- Onion, chopped, 1 cup
- Beating 4 eggs
- A delicate creme
- 235 milliliters (1 cup) of fat-free milk
- 2 teaspoons baking powder
- Nutmeg, to taste, 1/8 teaspoon
- Size: 12 oz (340 g) Tender, frozen spinach, defrosted and minced
- A total of 4 ounces (115 grams) of sliced mushrooms
- 1 cup shredded Monterey Cheddar Jack
- Shredded, 1 cup (115 g) to grate some Cheddar cheese
- One pre-made pie crust

Procedure:

- Throw bacon and onion in a skillet to cook together. Stir up the bacon. Join everything in a huge bowl.
- Place in quiche skillet with pie outside layer.
- Place in the broiler and heat for 50 minutes at 325 F.
- Ten minutes of rest time is suggested prior to serving.

As a portion:

- 4g-salt;
- 19g-protein;
- 22g-fat
- 2g-sugar;
- 297mg-sodium,
- 300mg-potassium,

7.   Baked Spinach

It's perfect for breakfast, but it also pairs well with other proteins like chicken and steak.

Ingredients:

- A package of frozen spinach weighing 10 ounces (280 grams)
- A dozen eggs, whisked
- 2 cups (450 g) (450 g) In the form of cottage cheese
- a quarter cup (55 grams) of unsalted butter, melted
- flour, 6 tablespoons (48 g)
- One tenth of a pound (283 g) Cubes of Cheddar cheese

Procedure:

- To set up the broiler, set the temperature to 350F.
- Spinach ought to be cooked concurring bundle guidelines, then depleted and crushed dry.
- Join everything in a 9-by-13-inch (23-by-33-centimeter) skillet.
- Planning time is one hour in the broiler.

As a portion:

- 143g-water
- 423-calories
- 20g-protein,
- 29g-fat
- 10g-carbohydrates,

8.   Breakfast Stuffed with Black Beans and Spinach

Very similar in speed to fast food, this will give you a refreshing change of pace to start the day with 12 grams of fiber to boot.

Ingredients:

- 1 egg
- Cornmeal, about one-fourth cup (35 g)
- 1/4 cup (20 g) (20 g) oats, rolled
- Two teaspoons of oat bran
- Wheat germ, 2 teaspoons
- A toasted wheat cereal, such Wheaten, 2 tablespoons (about 18 g)
- Baking soda, one teaspoon
- Baking powder, half a teaspoon
- One-tenth of a teaspoon of vanilla essence
- 1/2 a cup (355 g) of fat-free milk

- 2 whites of eggs

Procedures:

- Start the cooker temperature up to 350F (180 degrees Celsius, or gas mark 4).
- Scramble the combined egg and egg white in a shallow pan.
- Using a spatula, combine the following five ingredients.
- Fill the tortilla with the ingredients.
- Using a nonstick vegetable oil spray, wrap the two sides over securely and set the roller side down on a cooking sheet.

As a portion:

- 320g-water,
- 363-calories
- 26g-protein,
- 13g-total-fat
- 39g-carbohydrates,
- 12g-fiber,
- 4g-sugar,

9. Burrito for breakfast

Everything about this breakfast burrito is delicious. It's also convenient to grab on the fly.

Ingredients:

- 2 ounces of chorizo (55 g), coarsely chopped
- Onion, diced, half cup
- Red pepper,
- a single whole wheat tortilla
- one egg, beaten
- Sour cream, to taste, 2 teaspoons (30 g)
- 0.04 kilograms (55 g) Monterey Shredded or crumbled Jack cheese

Procedure:

- Set stove temperature to 400F (200C, gas mark 6).
- Cook the chorizo, onion, and chime powder in a little heater over moderate intensity until the meat is presently not pink. Gather the fat and channel it.
- Enclose the tortilla by the clammy kitchen towel and put it on a baking container.
- The tortilla needs something like 3 minutes in the broiler. Mix the sharp cream and egg together.

As a portion:

- 710-calories

- 39g-protein;
- 51g-fat
- 25g-carbohydrates
- 531mg-phosphorus,
- 539mg-calcium,
- Four-milligrams-iron,

10. Pancakes Made with Whole Wheat Flour and Buttermilk

Excellent pancakes in the classic style. Like the breakfasts my grandma used to make.

Ingredients:

- 120 grams (1 cup) whole wheat pastry flour
- A pinch of baking powder
- Cinnamon, Quarter Teaspoonful
- 1.25 ounces (64 ml) buttermilk
- 2 eggs
- 45 milliliters (3 tablespoons) of canola oil

Procedure:

- Combine the dry components. The liquids, excluding the oil, should be mixed together. Combine the two ingredients together. There will be some bumps.
- A cast-iron skillet should be heated with oil. Divide the batter in half and pour into the pan. Stir every one to two minutes, or until you see bubbles form.

11. Crepes made with cornmeal

A classic breakfast dish that has been around for a long time. So, you think I keep bringing it up because food was better back then?

Ingredients:

- Water to boil, one cup (235 ml)
- 3/4 cup of cornmeal (105 grams)
- 1 1/4 cups (295 ml) (295 ml) buttermilk
- 2 eggs
- 120 grams pastry flour
- A Baking Soda Sodium Bicarbonate Mixture, 1/4 Tea
- 1/4 cup of canola oil (60 ml)

Procedure:

- Whisk cornmeal and water together in a large bowl until the slightly thickened. Eggs and buttermilk should be combined. Stir the flour, baking soda, and baking powder together. Add to the slurry of cornmeal..

- Mix with some canola oil. Griddle it up!

12. Granola Pancakes

These pancakes are fantastic; they're heartier than average pancakes and packed with flavor. Make sure to add the apple topping described in Chapter 23.

Ingredients:

- Two teaspoons of oat bran
- Wheat germ, 2 teaspoons
- A toasted wheat cereal, such Wheaten, 2 tablespoons (about 18 g)
- Baking soda, one teaspoon
- Baking powder, half a teaspoon
- One-tenth of a teaspoon of vanilla essence
- 1/2 a cup (355 g) of fat-free milk
- 2 whites of eggs

Procedure:

- Add all the dry ingredients together. Batter is ready when milk and vanilla are added. Pancakes with a thicker batter will be just that. Place aside for half an hour of downtime.
- Be sure to whip the egg whites until they stiffen into peaks.
- After the resting period, gently incorporate into the batter.
- Put by the spoonful onto a hot griddle, and keep turning until the bubbles pop.
- Toss and turn until meat is done. Due to the thicker batter, these pancakes need extra time in the oven.

13. Skillet Pancakes Made with Oat Bran

I don't see why morning meals have to be bland and full of empty calories. If you're bored, you should try these pancakes.

Ingredients:

- 100 grams (1 cup) oat bran
- One-third of a cup (60 grams) of flour
- Sugar, 2 teaspoons' worth (9 g)
- 9 g (2 tablespoons) of baking powder
- 1.25 ounces (235 ml) of fat-free milk
- Canola oil, one tablespoon (around 15 ml)
- Egg white, one

Procedure:

- Preheat griddle in the middle of the oven. Lightly coat with vegetable oil spray that does not stick. Combine the first four ingredients by stirring. Whisk together the other ingredients, then add them to the oat bran mixture.

- Place batter by the spoonful on the griddle and flip the meat.

14. Cinnamon and oat bran

On a cold winter day, nothing beats a stack of these savory pancakes to warm your belly. The good news is that these pancakes are also far healthier than your average kind.

Ingredients:

- 3/4 cup (75 g) (75 g) grain oats
- Baking powder, half a teaspoon
- a half a teaspoon of cinnamon
- A Baking Soda Sodium Bicarbonate Mixture, 1/4 Tea
- 1.25 ounces (64 ml) buttermilk

Procedure:

- Place the dried ingredients into a mixing bowl of a medium size and mix them together using a whisk. It is necessary to take the dish away from the table.
- In a low-sided bowl or container, cream and butter should be combined and stirred. Stir until the liquid and dry ingredients are nearly completely combined. Incorporate the chopped pecans, then give the mixture a thorough swirl.
- To prepare on a sizzling griddle. To make four medium-sized pancakes, you'll need a quarter cup of batter.

15. Pancakes made with oats

As an alternative to the typical Sunday morning breakfast.

Ingredients:

- Reduced-fat milk, 1 1/4 cups (285 ml)
- 1 cup (80 g) (80 g) Instant Oatmeal
- 2 eggs
- Whole wheat flour, about half a cup (60 g)
- brown sugar, one tablespoon's worth (15 g)
- Cinnamon, one teaspoon (2.3 g)

Procedure:

- Mix the milk and oats together and let sit for 5 minutes. Eggs should be added and the mixture should be stirred well. When you've added all the other ingredients, whisk them in until they're evenly distributed.
- Place the pancakes on a hot griddle and flip until bubbles appear on the top and burst. To finish cooking the other side of the pancakes, turn them over.

16.   Pancakes made with bananas

I created this recipe while looking for a breakfast option that would make use of some overripe bananas. They're delicious on their own, and you won't need any extra sweetener (though a dusting of powdered sugar never hurts).

Ingredients:

- 125 grams (1 cup) of flour
- Suggested Ingredients Sugar, 1 Tablespoon (13 g)
- 14 grams of baking powder, or 1 tablespoon
- The equivalent of half a cup (120 ml) of skim milk
- 1 egg
- Canola oil, one tablespoon (around 15 ml)
- Banana, one cup (about 225 grams) cut

Procedure:

- Mix the dried items flour & powder together. Blend with the oil, egg, and milk together.
- Banana should be added to the mix. The flour and milk combination should be added simultaneously. Mix till smooth but some lumps remain.
- A nonstick vegetable oil spray should be used on a heated griddle before adding roughly half cup of batter.
- Brown the bottom (when bubbles appear and burst on top) before on with cooking. Cook the second side until it reaches the desired doneness. Gather the leftover batter and start again.

17.   Pancakes topped with apples

Excellent weekend breakfast, this (or maybe when you are snowed in). Like apple fritters, except the pancakes are fried with the syrup to fully absorb the sweet taste.

Ingredients:

- Four ounces (about 440 grams) of sliced apples
- Biscuit Baking Mix, 1 1/2 Cups (192 G)
- 1 cup (235 ml) (235 ml) watered-down milk
- 2 eggs
- a half a teaspoon of cinnamon
- A Nutmeg Pinch

Procedure:

- Throw some apples, some syrup, and some butter into a hot pan. After around 25 minutes of cooking, the vegetables should be soft but still have some bite to them. In the meanwhile, whisk the remaining ingredients together.

- Making a slotted spoon, scoop the apples out of the pan and add them to the batter. Apples should be carefully folded in until they are completely coated.
- Roll the apple slices in the batter and place them on the hot griddle that has been rolled with vegetable oil polish to prevent sticking. Grill it until the outsides are browned. Flip pancakes once.

18. High-Protein Blueberry Pancakes

Try these pancakes the next time you want a hearty meal but don't want to sacrifice taste for health.

Ingredients:

- 4 eggs
- 1 cup (225 g) (225 g) Cheese made from curds and whey
- 1 gm grain germ
- Instant Oatmeal
- 1.5 teaspoons (28 ml) olive oil
- blueberries, one cup (145 g)

Procedure:

- Blend together everything except the blueberries. Add blueberries and stir. Serve on a hot griddle or skillet sprayed with nonstick vegetable oil. Drop by the tablespoonful.

19. Crepe Baked in the Oven

To make, just combine all of the ingredients, then bake and serve. A perfect breakfast option for the weekend.

Ingredients:

- 3 eggs
- Whole wheat pastry flour, to taste, about 1/2 cup (60 g).
- The equivalent of half a cup (120 ml) of skim milk
- a quarter cup (55 g) of unsalted butter, cut into
- 2 tbsp (or 26 g) of sugar
- Toast the almonds and use them to fill 2 teaspoons (18 g)
- The juice of two lemons, around 30 milliliters

Procedure:

- For best results, use a medium-speed electric mixer to whip the eggs. Beat in the flour gradually until a smooth dough forms.
- Mix in the butter with 2 tablespoons of milk until the batter is smooth. The batter should be poured into a nonstick 10-inch (25-cm) pan.
- Cook until pancake is puffy and golden brown, about 15 minutes at 400f temp.

- Toss with sugar and toasted nuts. To melt the remaining butter, mix in the lemon juice. Serve on a heated pancake.

20. French Toast

Pancakes in the German manner are prepared in a single huge pan and then sliced into individual portions.

Ingredients:

- Pastry flour, whole wheat: 1 1/2 cups (180 g)
- 1 1/2 cups (35 ml) (35 ml) watered-down milk
- Incorporate 4 eggs with a little beating.
- Melted unsalted butter, about a quarter cup (55 g)
- Approximately 1 cup (170 g) of sliced strawberries

Procedure:

- Making a slotted spoon, scoop the apples out of the pan and add them to the batter. Apples should be carefully folded in until they are completely coated.
- Roll the apple slices in the batter and place them on the hot griddle that has been rolled with vegetable oil polish to prevent sticking. Grill it until the outsides are browned. Flip pancakes once.

21. Waffles made with wheat flour

These are great with breakfast, but we also prefer them for supper with a savory topping, such as chicken a la king.

Ingredients:

- 2 cups of whole wheat pastry flour (about 240 grams)
- Baking powder, about 4 teaspoons' worth (18 g)
- Honey, about 2 teaspoons' worth (40 grams)
- 1 3/4 cups (410 ml) (410 ml) watered-down milk
- 60 milliliters (4 tablespoons) of canola oil
- 2 eggs

Procedure:

- Mixer the dried items in a mixing bowl. Add the rest of the ingredients and stir. Separating the eggs makes the waffles lighter.
- Cook until pancake is puffy and golden brown, about 15 minutes at 400f temp.
- Toss with sugar and toasted nuts. To melt the remaining butter, mix in the lemon juice. Serve on a heated waffle.

22.   Cups of orange juice for breakfast

The process is fast and simple. However, it is more than simply grapefruit and oranges thanks to the inclusion of the grapes and almonds.

Ingredients:

- Four Grapefruits
- Two hundred and fifty grams (2 cups) of green grapes without the seeds.
- 1/2 tsp. sugar 2 oranges, sliced (27 g) Almonds, sliced thinly, roasted

Procedure:

- Slicing grapefruits in half is a good idea. Take off the insides and the membrane, but leave the shells alone.
- Just toss the grapes, oranges, and grapefruit slices together. Chill. Just before serving, toss some nuts into the fruit bowl. Fill grapefruit halves with the fruit mixture.

23.   Fruits dipped in an Orange Cream Sauce

It's OK to serve this dip to guests at a social gathering, but it's also a good idea to serve it to your own family, since it contains many healthy ingredients.

Ingredients:

- The equivalent of one cup of sour cream (230 grams)
- 1.5 teaspoons (30 g) Brown sugar, tightly compressed
- 15 milliliters (1 tablespoon) of orange juice
- To a teaspoon, orange peel
- Pineapple chunks, one cup's worth (165 grams)
- 1-cup (195 g) orange parts
- Kiwifruit, sliced (1 cup/177 g)
- 145 g or 1 cup of strawberries

Procedure:

- All of the ingredients, excluding the fruit, should be mixed in a medium-sized serving dish. Keep chilled for at least two hours after covering.
- Put some fresh fruit on skewers and serve it with the dip.

24. Fruit Sauce

A basic, raw fruit sauce. Spread this on top of some whole wheat pancakes for a special treat.

Ingredients:

- Apple juice
- Totally four cored and peeled apples
- 2 cups (300 g) (300 g) bananas cut into slices
- 1 pear, cored and sliced in half
- 1/2 teaspoon ginger
- The equivalent of one teaspoon of nutmeg

Procedure:

- Fruits and apple juice should be blended together. To blend to a uniform consistency. Once that's done, stir in the seasonings.

25. Bars for Breakfast

These are a healthy alternative to store-bought granola bars, and they're great for grabbing before hitting the road in the morning.

Ingredients:

- 1 cup Instant Oatmeal
- a half a teaspoon of cinnamon
- 1 egg
- 14 cup (60 g) apple sauce
- Honey, about a quarter cup's worth (85 g)
- There should be 3 tablespoons (45 g) Sugar, brown
- Canola oil, to taste, about 2 teaspoons (28 ml)
- Unsalted sunflower seeds, about a quarter cup (36 g)
- 30 g (one-fourth cup) of chopped walnuts
- Dried fruits, around 7 ounces

Procedure:

- For best results, preheat the broiler to 325 ° F. (170 degrees C, gas mark 3). Prepare a square baking dish, 9 inches (23 centimeters) in size, by lining it with aluminum foil.
- Nonstick vegetable oil shower ought to be splashed on the foil. Mix the oats, flour, cereal, and cinnamon in an enormous bowl. Put in the egg, fruit purée, honey, earthy colored sugar, and oil. Set up everything in a decent, even combination.
- Blend in the pecans, dried organic product, and sunflower seeds. Coat the base and the sides of the container with the combination. Leave in the broiler for 30 minutes, or until the

edges are firm and brilliant. Set to the side to cool. To eliminate from the dish, snatch a sheet of foil and use it as a handle. Make bars and keep in the ice chest.

26. Banana-flavored cereal bar cookies

Oatmeal and bananas make a delicious duo. Even better, you can have these cookies for breakfast or as a midday snack and they'll be delicious either way.

Ingredients:

- 3 eggs
- 3 cups pastry flour made from whole wheat
- 1/2 cups Instant Oatmeal
- Baking soda, one teaspoon
- bananas, mashed, 2 cups (450 grams)
- Chopped pecans, one cup's worth (around 110 grams)

Procedure:

- Join the sugar and shortening in a bowl. Mix in the eggs well. Joining the flour, baking pop, nutmeg, and cinnamon by filtering is the initial step. Mix oats into the shortening. To the flour combination, add the squashed bananas in three options.
- Those walnuts should be slashed and added. Scatter on a baking sheet showered with nonstick vegetable oil splash. 12-15 minutes at 375 degrees F.

27. Carrot-Chip Biscuits for Breaky

Another convenient breakfast food to grab and go.

Ingredients:

- Grated Carrots: 1 Cup (110 G)
- Fat-free plain yogurt, about 1/2 cup (115 g)
- 60 grams (1/4 cup) of dark sugar
- Canola oil, to taste, about 2 teaspoons (28 ml)
- 12 cup milk 14 teaspoon vanilla essence (220 g) dried fruits, chopped
- 1 1/2 cups (180 g) (180 g) pastry flour made from whole wheat
- Grape-Nuts or any similar crisp wheat-barley cereal, about 1/4 cup (29 g)
- A pinch of baking powder

Procedure:

- Prepare a square baking dish, 9 inches (23 centimeters) in size, by lining it with aluminum foil.
- Consolidate the carrot, yogurt, sugar, oil, vanilla, and dates in a medium bowl and blend well. Stand by fifteen minutes prior to endeavoring. Mix in the other dry fixings by blending.

- Spread the batter out on baking sheets using a tablespoon, leaving about 4 centimeters (1 1/2 inches) between each ball. Miniature cookies can be made by reducing the ingredients to the level of a teaspoon's drops. If you touch the top of the cookies after 15 minutes, they should bounce back. Cool.

28. Cookies for Breaking the Fast

This is a convenient option for a quick morning meal. They're on the softer side, but they're easily transportable and have no fat.

Ingredients:

- Bananas that have been mashed
- Fat-free plain yogurt, about 1/2 cup (115 g)
- 60 grams (1/4 cup) of dark sugar
- Canola oil, to taste, about 2 teaspoons (28 ml)
- 12 cup milk 14 teaspoon vanilla essence (220 g) dried fruits, chopped
- Dried cranberries, about half a cup (75 grams)
- One Tablespoon (5 ml) vanilla
- One Tablespoon (2.3 g) cinnamon
- . Suggested **Ingredients:** Sugar, 1 Tablespoon (13 g)
- 50 grams (half a cup) of chopped pecans

Procedure:

- In order to prepare the broiler, set the temperature to 180 ° C. (gas level 4) which is equivalent to 350 ° f Fahrenheit. Pour everything together in a dish and mix it up well. If it is not too much of an inconvenience for you, please wait for about five minutes before using this mixture.
- Using a spoonful, transfer the batter to a cookie sheet that has been greased. After baking, let it fifteen to twenty minutes to cool down before handling it.

29. Crispy Topping for Oatmeal

You can use it on everything from porridge and toast to fruit and yogurt to pancakes and waffles and even French toast.

Ingredients:

- Melted unsalted butter, about a quarter cup (55 g)
- Fat-free plain yogurt, about 1/2 cup (115 g)
- 60 grams (1/4 cup) of dark sugar
- Canola oil, to taste, about 2 teaspoons (28 ml)
- 12 cup milk 14 teaspoon vanilla essence (220 g) dried fruits, chopped
- One Tablespoon of Orange Peel, Grated

- a half a teaspoon of cinnamon

Procedure:

- Combine the remaining ingredients. Ten to twelve minutes in the oven should provide a golden crispness. Stir. Keep refrigerated for up to three months after cooling.

30. Granola

If you're cautious about what you buy and study the labels, you may find certain cereals that are good for you. A granola that is both healthier and more delicious than this homemade kind is unlikely to be discovered.

Ingredients:

- 6 cups oats, rolled
- To make 6 servings of rolled wheat,
- Sunflower seeds, about 2 cups (290 grams)
- Four Ounces (113 g) oily seeds often used in Asian cooking
- Toasted peanuts, 2 cups (190 g)
- 3 cups coconut
- 1 cup grain germ
- 1 1/2 cups olive oil
- Honey, one cup's worth (340 grams)
- Molasses, 1/2 cup (170 g)
- 2 teaspoons (15 ml) Pure vanilla essence
- 1 cup (145 g) raisins

Procedure:

- In a huge dish, consolidate the dry fixings in general (with the exception of the raisins). Quit mulling over everything for the present. Mix oil, honey, molasses, and vanilla over low intensity, then, at that point, add to dry fixings. Cover baking sheets with the combination.

- For 30-40 minutes at 350°F (180°C, gas mark 4), until softly cooked. Continuously be blending to get an equivalent cooking. Take out the broiler and blend in with some dried organic product, such raisins.

31. Super Scrambled Eggs on Toast

Ingredients

- Egg whites
- Ezekiel or whole meal bread
- Onion
- Yellow peppers
- White mushrooms

- Garlic
- Parsley
- Olive oil

Procedures:

- Whisk together the milk, eggs, and cumin in a bowl to combine the ingredients.
- Cooking spray should be applied to the pan before it is placed over medium heat. Simmer the ingredients for a few minutes.
- Approximately after a few minutes, stir in some low-fat cheese, red peppers that have been diced, and black beans to the omelet.
- When everything is in place, fold the omelct in half and let it cook for another minute or two.
- After removing from the skillet, serve with the salsa and the chopped coriander.

32. Banana And Almond Muscle Oatmeal

Ingredients

- Rolled oats
- milk
- Whey protein
- almonds
- peanut butter
- Banana

Procedures:

- Place the oats and milk with a reduced fat content in a big bowl, give it a good stir, and then put it in the microwave for a couple of minutes.
- Combine the oats with the chopped almonds, peanut butter, and whey protein, and then add the banana, which has been diced.

33. Protein Powered Pancakes

Ingredients:

- Egg whites
- Rolled oats
- Flaxseed oil
- Cinnamon
- Stevia

Procedures:

- In a blender, combine the oats with the rest of the ingredients and mix until smooth. The batter for your pancakes is now ready.

- Before placing the pan over medium heat, coat it with cooking spray.
- Transfer about one fifth of the pancake batter to the pan and allow it to cook for one to two minutes. Cooking for a further thirty seconds after you have flipped the pancake.
- When it is finished cooking, remove your delicious pancake.
- Continue with the rest of the batter in the same way.
- Accompany the dish with the fruit of your choosing.

34. Fried Omelets

Ingredients

- Turkey
- Eggs
- Spinach
- Kale
- Olive oil
- Cheese

Procedures:

- Place the eggs in a bowl and use a whisk to mix them until they are uniform in color.
- Grab a pan and set it over medium heat while you heat up half of the oil. After that, throw in the ground turkey, greens, and cheese, and keep the heat on for another five or six minutes.
- In a separate pan, heat the remaining quantity of olive oil, add the eggs, and continue to cook the combination for about four minutes.
- After adding the turkey mixture to the eggs in the pan, sprinkle some baby spinach over the top of the omelet, and then fold it in half to eat.
- Keep stirring the mixture every two to three minutes as it cooks.
- Arrange the meal, and then serve it to the guests.

35. Aesthetic Asparagus Frittata

Ingredients

- Asparagus
- Broccoli
- Eggs
- Parsley
- Chives
- Olive oil
- Milk
- Salt And Pepper

Procedures:

- In a bowl, break the eggs, add the milk, and season with salt and pepper, then mix everything together.
- Place the broccoli florets in a covered pan and cook them over medium heat for around four to five minutes. Put put one side for now.
- The next step is to heat the oil in the same skillet. After the asparagus, parsley, and chives have been chopped, add them to the pan and sauté them for around two to three minutes over medium heat.
- Pour the egg mixture into the skillet along with the broccoli, and spread it out so that it covers the whole bottom of the pan.
- Continue to cook for another three to four minutes, or until the eggs are firm all the way through.
- Place the skillet on the grill for about two minutes, or until the top has a golden-browncolor (this step is optional).
- Arrange the food and serve it.

36. Chipotle Pumpkin Soup

Ingredients:

- One medium butternut squash, unsliced andslice into cubes shapes
- One and a half cup feta cheese, crumbled
- One and a half cup butternuts, sliced
- Half tsp dried thyme
- Two cups vegetables
- One cup farro, uncooked
- One onion, chopped
- Two tsp olive oil
- One and a half tsp pepper
- One and a half tsp salt

Procedures:

- Combine oil within the immediate pot cooker and arranged the container on heating mode.
- Supplement onion and cook for 3-4 minutes.
- Combine farro and bake for more extra minutes.
- Add stock and mix thoroughly.
- Put the cooking rack above the farro batter and set squash on theshelf.
- Season with black pepper, flavorings, and spice, salt.
- Lock pot with top and bake on raised for 8-10 minutes.
- Discharge pressure using the quick removal method, then loosen the cover.
- Get spoon squash inside a container.

- Supplement farro ingredients and mix thoroughly.
- Moisten with cheese and butternuts.
- Serve and enjoy the meal.

Nutritional info:
- Calories: 225-230;
- Carbohydrates: 18-20g;
- Protein: 10-12g;
- Fat: 13-15g;
- Sugar: 4.4-5g;
- Sodium: 799-800mg

37. Stuffed Mushrooms

Ingredients:
- One and a half cup washed rice.
- Two tbsp curry flour
- One cup medium MUSHROOM head, separate into florets.
- One tbsp turmeric
- Olive or plant oil
- Butter
- One cup BROWN-BEAN
- Fresh Cheese
- Two tsp vinegar
- Two tbsp turmeric
- Chili powder
- Condiments
- Curry masala
- Two tsp olive oil
- Three cups drinking water
- One and a half tsp salt

Procedures:
- Discharge one cup of freshwater inside the instant cooker pot.
- Combine MUSHROOMS head florets inside the immediate container steamship container.
- Lock container with cover and heat on standard extraordinary for one or more minutes.
- Relief pressure utilizing the immediate discharge process, then remove the cover.
- Transfer the MUSHROOMS from the container and put it on a recipe.
- Discharge liquid from the immediate cooker pot.
- Combine olive-oil inside the container and arranged the container on heat method.

Chapter 4

Main Dishes: Vegetables

38. Portobello Mushrooms on the Grill

In place of beef, try this easy dish for grilled portobellos.

Ingredients:

- Four stemmed and cleaned portobello mushroom caps

- 1/4 cup (60 ml) (60 ml) Vinegar of Modena (or Balsamic)

- Add 1 tablespoon (15 ml) of olive oil.

- One Tablespoon (0.7 g) a kind of basil that is normally dried

- Dried oregano, one teaspoon (1 g)

- A Half Teaspoon (1.5 g) garlic, minced

- 4.08 ounces (115 g) lower in fat Cubed Provolone Cheese

Procedure:

Arrange the mushroom tops, smooth side up, in a pie plate. Vinegar, oil, basil, oregano, and garlic should all be combined. Toss the mushrooms with the liquid. Allow to sit out for 15 minutes, rotating twice, at room temperature. Turn grill heat up to medium-high. Brush oil onto the grill. Grill the mushrooms, and save aside some of the marinate to use later as a basting sauce. Cook for 5–8 minutes on each side, or until cooked, on a hot grill. Spread the marinade on a brush and use it liberally. Grill for another 2 minutes after adding cheese.

39. Hawaii's Famous Portobello Burgers

Although portobello mushrooms are a relatively new addition to our diet, they have rapidly become a fan favorite. You won't even need meat in this sandwich because of how tasty it is.

Ingredients:

- 2 stemless, cleaned portobello mushrooms

- Two Tablespoons (30 ml) To make Dick's Low Sodium Teriyaki Sauce (recipe on page 25), follow these steps:

- A half-pineapple

- 2 low-fat slices Cheese made from Monterey Jack sheep

- It's only two leaves of lettuce.

- A few of tomatoes

- Two hamburger buns

- 2 teaspoons (14 g) reduced-fat mayonnaise

Procedure:

- Gently and artfully place the exquisite mushrooms in a harmonious formation, ensuring they grace the surface of the wide, shallow dish in a single, captivating layer. For a truly tantalizing flavor infusion, generously coat your ingredients with a luscious teriyaki sauce, allowing it to permeate every nook and cranny.

- Allow this delectable concoction to work its magic as you patiently wait for a mere 15 minutes, allowing the flavors to meld together in perfect harmony. Gently caress the mushroom and pineapple slices over the flickering embers, allowing them to surrender to the heat until they reach a state of tender succulence. Gently crown the succulent grilled mushrooms with a luscious layer of cheese, allowing the heat to work its magic and gracefully melt the cheese into a creamy, indulgent delight.

- Continue grilling for a few more minutes, ensuring that every bite is a harmonious symphony of flavors. Indulge in the art of burger construction, where each layer is meticulously crafted to create a symphony of flavors. Begin this culinary masterpiece by delicately placing the foundation of the burger - the bottom buns. On this canvas, carefully arrange a bed of crisp lettuce, vibrant tomatoes, earthy mushrooms, and a surprising touch of sweetness with succulent pineapple.

- Gently spread a luscious layer of creamy mayonnaise atop the crown of each delectable bun, ensuring an even distribution that will tantalize the taste buds.

40. Vegetable Curry from the Caribbean

A vegetarian curry dish with a moderate heat level. Cayenne pepper may be added to taste.

Ingredients:

- Add 1 tablespoon (15 ml) of olive oil.
- 1 cup (160 g) finely sliced onion
- A half-pineapple
- 2 low-fat slices Cheese made from Monterey Jack sheep
- It's only two leaves of lettuce.
- A few of tomatoes
- Two hamburger buns
- 2 teaspoons (14 g) reduced-fat mayonnaise
- a single teaspoon of coriander
- 1/4 of a teaspoon of turmeric
- Fifteenth of a teaspoon of chili pepper
- A half-pineapple
- 2 low-fat slices Cheese made from Monterey Jack sheep

- It's only two leaves of lettuce.
- A few of tomatoes
- Two hamburger buns
- 2 teaspoons (14 g) reduced-fat mayonnaise
- Hard-boiled eggs x 3 (cut in half)
- 3 cups (495 g) (495 g) Fried Rice
- Sliced radishes (about 6)
- sliced scallions, about a quarter cup (25 grams)
- a half a cup of fresh cilantro, chopped
- Nuts, chopped; about a quarter cup (37 g)

Procedure:

- Flush the oil in the pan. Cook the onion, garlic, and apple until they are tender in a skillet. Meld together the curry, lemon peel, ginger, coriander, turmeric, and cayenne. Combine with the onions and stir well. Mix in the dried fruits and beans, including the kidney beans that have not been drained.

- Simmer, covered, for 5 minutes. Take it off the heat and mix with some yogurt. Cover the rice with the egg halves. Put some curry on it. Use radishes, scallions, cilantro, and peanuts as garnishes.

41. Spiced Tomato and Bean Curry

You could serve this as a side with grilled chicken or pig loin, or eat it on its own as a vegetarian main course. When that's the case, it's best to eat it with rice or pita bread.

Ingredients:

- Canola oil, one tablespoon (around 15 ml)
- Mustard seed, about 1 teaspoon's worth (3.7 g)
- Cumin seeds, one teaspoonful (2.5 g)
- Onions: 1 cup (about 160 grams) chopped
- Fresh ginger, peeled and diced to equal 1 tablespoon (6 g)
- Chopped garlic, half a teaspoon (1.5 g)
- Cans containing four servings (720 grams) Tomates without sel
- 2 cups (450 grams) of drained and washed kidney beans
- 2 grams of curry powder, or one teaspoon

Procedure:

- Beat an egg with some sour cream, some water, and some Italian spice until light and airy. Mushrooms, onion, and green bell pepper should be sautéed until the onion is tender.

- When the pan or skillet is hot, spray it with vegetable oil spray and add the egg mixture. When cooking, lift the sides to let the raw egg seep below.

42. Curried Tofu

This has to be one of the quickest and easiest vegetarian dishes out there. The curry should be served over rice and topped with preferred seasonings.

Ingredients:

- 12 ounces (340 g) firm tofu, rinsed and cubed 3 tablespoons (45 ml) olive oil, divided

- Cumin seeds, one teaspoonful (2.5 g)

- Onions: 1 cup (about 160 grams) chopped

- Fresh ginger, peeled and diced to equal 1 tablespoon (6 g)

- Chopped garlic, half a teaspoon (1.5 g)

- Cans containing four servings (720 grams) Tomates without sel

- 2 cups (450 grams) of drained and washed kidney beans

- 2 grams of curry powder, or one teaspoon

Procedure:

Beat an egg with some sour cream, some water, and some Italian spice until light and airy. Mushrooms, onion, and green bell pepper should be sautéed until the onion is tender. When the pan or skillet is hot, spray it with vegetable oil spray and add the egg mixture. When cooking, lift the sides to let the raw egg seep below.

To a plate, please. Toss the zucchini and mushrooms in the remaining oil and stir-fry them until they are soft. Cook the milk and curry powder together until the mixture has thickened a little. Blend in the tofu and heat through.

43. Pizza omelet

The Pizza Omelet is the perfect solution for those times when you're craving pizza but don't want to spend the time or effort cooking it from scratch. The omelet is large enough to serve as a main course for two people.

Ingredients:

- 4 eggs

- Amount: 2 tablespoons (30 g) fat-free sour cream

- The equivalent of 2 teaspoons (30 ml) of water

- A Half Teaspoon (0.4 g) Spices from Italy

- Thinly sliced mushrooms, 1/2 cup (35 g)

- Ingredients 14 cup (40 g) sliced onion 14 cup (37 g) coarsely chopped green bell pepper

- Spaghetti with warmed sauce (1/4 cup, 60 ml) 2 ounces (55 g) of shredded part-skim mozzarella

Procedure:

- Beat an egg with some sour cream, some water, and some Italian spice until light and airy. Mushrooms, onion, and green bell pepper should be sautéed until the onion is tender. When the pan or skillet is hot, spray it with vegetable oil spray and add the egg mixture.

- When cooking, lift the sides to let the raw egg seep below. Near the end of cooking time, spread the veggies over half the omelet and fold the other half over the top. Put it on a platter. Melted cheese and hot sauce go well together.

44. Omelet with Ricotta

With a side salad and some crusty bread, this makes a great summer meal. Vegetables are optional.

Ingredients:

- 4 eggs

- Powdered garlic, equivalent to a quarter teaspoon (0.8 g)

- Pepper, black, one-fourth teaspoon (0.5 g)

- Reduced-fat ricotta cheese, about a half cup (125 g)

- 30 milliliters (2 tablespoons) of olive oil

Procedure:

- Blend the ricotta, garlic powder, and pepper into the beaten eggs. Get an omelet pan or skillet hot and add the oil. Add the beaten eggs and stir to disperse them evenly. When the egg is almost done, raise the edge to let the uncooked egg flow below. Cover and cook on low heat until done.

- Quiche with Tomatoes and Basil

- Awesome vegan quiche. You can heat it in a covering in the event that you wish, yet we believe it's perfect without.

45. Tarte à la Artichaut

Great veggie lover dish with an Italian taste.

Ingredients:

- 3 eggs

- Relaxed cream cheddar including chives, 3 ounces (85 g)

- Garlic powder, around 3/4 teaspoon

- 1/4 teaspoon dark pepper

- Destroyed mozzarella cheddar, 1 1/2 cups (225 g)

- 1 cup (250 g) (250 g) cream cheddar

- 1/2 cup (115 g) (115 g) low-fat mayo

- 1 can artichoke hearts

- Arranged chickpeas, one cup (164 g)

- Dark olives, cut, 1/2 cup (50 g)

- 2 ounces (55 g) pimento, depleted and diced

- 2 teaspoons of slashed dried parsley

- 1 unbaked pie shell, around 9 inches (23 cm) in breadth

Procedure:

- Eggs ought to be sped in an enormous bowl. Consolidate cream cheddar, garlic powder, and dark pepper. Integrate the ricotta, mayonnaise, and 1 cup (150 g) of mozzarella. Eliminate and save 2 artichoke heart quarters. The leftover artichoke hearts ought to be hacked and added to the cheddar.

- Blend in the olives, pimiento, parsley, and chickpeas. Carry out mixture and fill it with the fixings. For 30 minutes, heat the broiler to 350 degrees Fahrenheit (180 degrees Celsius, gas mark

- Add the extra mozzarella and Parmesan on top.

- Keep baking for an additional 15 minutes, or until the middle is firm. Let represent 10 minutes. Artichokes, cut into fourths, for embellish.

46. Custard Pie

This recipe is perfect as a vegetarian main course; just add a salad to round out the meal.

Ingredients:

- 1 pound (450 g) feta cheese

- 4 eggs

- Powdered garlic, equivalent to a quarter teaspoon (0.8 g)

- Pepper, black, one-fourth teaspoon (0.5 g)

Procedure:

Make sure your oven is preheated to 375 degrees Fahrenheit (190 degrees Celsius, or gas mark 5). Use nonstick vegetable oil spray to grease a glass baking dish or oven-safe pan. Combine both types of cheese, then add the other ingredients (eggs, flour, milk, and pepper) and mix until everything is evenly distributed. Pour the batter into the prepared \span. To get a beautiful brown and set result, bake for 40 minutes. Divide into triangles.

47. Recipe for Whole Wheat Apple Strata

This brunch is now customary on Christmas morning. Ham was originally called for in the recipe, but nobody seems to mind that it's been removed. Honestly, any kind of stale bread will do, but my personal preference is honey wheat. Apple pie filling may be substituted with canned apples, although the end product will be sweeter.

Ingredients:

- 6 cubed pieces of whole wheat bread 1 can of chopped apples (21 ounces, or 600 grams)

- 3 fluid ounces (85 g) lower in fat Shredded Cheddar Cheese

- 4 eggs

- 1/4 cup (60 ml) (60 ml) skim milk

Procedure:

- Put the bread in a square pan that's 9 inches (23 centimeters) on a side and sprayed with nonstick vegetable oil spray. Spread some apples on toast. Toss in some grated cheese. Eggs and milk may be mixed together and then poured over the bread. Put in the fridge overnight with plastic wrap over it.

- Turn the oven temperature up to 350 degrees Fahrenheit (180 degrees Celsius, or gas mark 4). To get a gently browned top and a set center, bake uncovered for 40 to 45 minutes.

Chapter 5

Side Dishes

48. Tomatoes with Stuffing

Stuffed tomatoes with rice, cheese, and vegetables are a tasty accompaniment to almost any meat.

Ingredients:

* Approximately 6 medium-sized tomatoes

* Two Tablespoons (28 ml) oil, olive

* 1/3 cup (33 g) (33 g) prepared with sliced celery

* Two Tablespoons (20 g) The Onion, chopped

* 2 cups (440 g) (440 g) A bowl of brown rice that's been cooked.

* 25 grams (0.1 cup) of freshly grated Parmesan

* Parsley, fresh, chopped: 1 tbsp.

* 1 tsp of dried basil

* Pepper, about one-eighth of a teaspoon

* (about) 18 tsp. of garlic

Procedure:

* Remove a little piece of the tomato's top. Leave caps out of it. Remove the pulp from the tomatoes by cutting it into small pieces and setting it aside. Drain the shells by setting them upside down on a paper towel.

* Prepare a pie dish or other circular baking dish, about 9 inches (23 cm) in diameter, by lightly oiling it. Put tomatoes on serving plate. Use aluminum foil to conceal. Set oven temperature to 350F (180C/gas 4).

49. Tomatoes Stuffed with Avocado

In particular, it goes well as a pre-meal snack or a side dish to a Mexican feast.

Ingredients:

- The equivalent of 4 tomatoes

- One avocado.

- Lemon Juice (About a Quarter of a

- Chili Powder, Half a Teaspoon

- Black bell pepper, diced, 1/4 cup (38 g)

- 1-milliliter portion of parsley

- Coriander, about one-fourth of a teaspoon

Procedure:

Remove the tomatoes' tops, and cut them open vertically. The meat should be reserved for another meal. Mix all of the ingredients together, including the mashed avocado. Stuff the tomato tops full of it.

50. Tempura-Battered Tomatoes

My mom used to prepare scalloped tomatoes all the time, but we never got around to eating them.

Ingredients:

- Due to our recent rediscovery, they are now a staple in our home.

- 30 milliliters (2 tablespoons) of olive oil

- Toss together 1/2 cup (80 g) chopped onion, 2 slices bread, and 3 cups (540 g) sliced tomatoes.

Procedure:

Increase the heat to 350 degrees Fahrenheit on the stovetop (180 degrees Celsius, or gas mark 4). In a container, warm the oil and sauté the onion until it has mellowed. Toss in some bread crumbs and give it a good toss to combine. Spread one layer of the tomatoes in a casserole dish that holds exactly 1 quart (946 ml). Spread half of the crumbs on top. Repeat \slayers. Cook for 30 minutes at 350 degrees.

51. Stuffed mushrooms with garlic sauce

Vegetables from Italy, roasted in the oven.

Ingredients:

- 30 milliliters (2 tablespoons) of olive oil

- Onion, cut into wedges (about 1/2 cup or 80 grams)

- Green bell pepper, about half a cup (75 g), diced into 1-inch (2.5-cm) chunks

- Plum tomato halves, about a quarter cup (45 g)

- Zucchini, about a half cup's worth (56 g), sliced into 1-inch (2.5-cm) rounds

- 30 grams (one half a cup) of sliced mushrooms

Procedure:

- Heat at 400F (200 degrees Celsius, or gas mark 6) for 10 minutes. In a zip-top plastic sack, blend the oil, garlic, basil, and oregano.
- Throw in the vegetables, including the onion, green ringer pepper, tomatoes, zucchini, and mushrooms. Splash some nonstick vegetable oil in a 9-by-13-inch (23-by-33-cm) broiling dish.
- Ensure the veggies are fanned out equitably in the dish. A generally pretty firm dinner may be achieved by cooking it for 20 minutes at 400 degrees.

52. Beans with Pearl Onions in Caramel Sauce

In place of the standard green bean casserole, serve this instead. It's less time-consuming to prepare, healthier, and more versatile than salty alternatives; and its sweet taste complements a wide range of dishes.

Ingredients:

- Green beans weighing 2 pounds (910 grams)

- a one pound (455 g) of pearl onions

- a third of a cup of unsalted butter (75 grams)

- Brown sugar, 1/2 cup (115 g)

Procedure:

- Get ready beans for steaming by putting them in a liner crate set over a pot of bubbling water. Put away following 15 minutes of covered steaming. Place onions in bubbling water for 3 minutes.
- Channel and wash switch cold water. Onions might be stripped and root closes cut off first. To steam onions, place a liner bin over dish of bubbling water.

- Wrap the bowl and steam for 5 minutes. The onions ought to be set to the side. Spread ought to be dissolved in a huge dish over medium intensity. Cook the sugar with consistent mixing until it starts to bubble. Throw in the onions and mix constantly for three minutes. Throw in the beans and intensity through while mixing frequently.

53. Soy Sauce with Sesame Green Beans

These beans would go well with any meal. They're delicious, healthy, and good for you since they contain no trans fats and are rich in fiber. So, really, what else could one want?

Ingredients:

- One Tablespoon of Sesame Seeds

- Green beans, about 1 pound (455 grams) (defrosted if frozen)

- 1/2 cup low sodium-reduced chicken stock

- Juice from 2 lemons, around 10 milliliters (2 tablespoons)

Procedure:

- For approximately three minutes over moderate heat, stirring the pan often, toast the sesame seeds until they are golden brown and popping. Include broth and green beans.

- Green beans will be done when most of the liquid has gone and they have been cooked for 7 to 8 minutes in a covered pan. Take it off the heat.

- Add some fresh lemon juice and mix it together before serving.

54. Limas with a Kick of Heat

This recipe was sent by a newsletter reader who included instructions for both baking and slow cooking. It's delicious on its own, or over brown rice, whole grain pasta, or vegetarian spaghetti, and can feed around 8 people.

Ingredients:

- Lima beans, about 2 cups (404 grams) of dry
- 4 glasses of water (940 ml)
- Mrs. Dash, 2 teaspoons really hot
- 1/2 milligram of garlic powder
- Onion, chopped, 1 cup (160 g)
- Half cup nicely diced green bell pepper
- 2 cups sliced Tomatoes in a pot with no salt added
- A measure of honey equal to 1 tablespoon (20 g)
- 1 tsp of dried basil
- 4 cup of dried thyme

Procedure:

• Lima beans that have been dried ought to be ready in the way determined by the maker. Add all the other things (with the exception of the lima beans) to a blending bowl and mix. Add lima beans circumspectly and blend.

• Covered baking dish of 2 to 4 quarts (2 to 4 L) limit is required.

• Involving a sluggish cooker as another option: In enough water to cover them, douse lima beans for 6 to 8 hours, then channel. Short-term (six to eight hours), slow stew beans in a covered sluggish cooker on low.

• Put the veggies and the other fixings into a sluggish cooker and cook on high for one hour. Add lima beans carefully and blend. Keep the intensity on low and cook until every one of the fluid has been retained.

55. Salad with Tomatoes and Green Beans

In a new and interesting direction, green beans. Pairs well with barbecued meat.

Ingredients:

• Green beans, about 1/2 pound (225 g)

• Add 1 tbsp (15 ml) of olive oil.

• sliced red pepper, about a quarter cup (38 g)

• 1 chopped onion (about 40 grams), 1 diced tomato (about 180 grams), 1/2 teaspoon salt (0.4 g) a kind of basil that is normally dried

• Half a teaspoon of dried rosemary (0.6 grams)

Procedure:

• To soften green beans, just boil them for a few minutes. Drain the water and store it. Saute red bell pepper and nion in oil till tender. Combine with tomatoes, herbs, and spices. Green beans should be heated completely and mixed together.

56. Recipe for Bean Salad

The result is a very standard three-bean salad. Low-sodium canned kidney beans or precooked dry beans may be substituted.

Ingredients:

• Cider vinegar, one and half cup (120 ml)

• sugar, half cup (50 g)

• 1/4 cup of oil (60 ml)

• Powdered garlic, equivalent to a quarter teaspoon (0.8 g)

- Pepper, black, one-fourth teaspoon (0.5 g)

- Green beans, 12 ounces (340 grams) thawed Yellow beans, 12 ounces (340 grams) thawed Wax beans

- beans, kidney, 1 cup (225 g) boiled

- Diced onion, about a quarter cup (40 grams)

- Diced green bell peppers, about a quarter cup (37 g)

Procedure:

In a pot, whisk together the vinegar, sugar, oil, garlic powder, and dark pepper. Dissolve the sugar by warming it. Green, yellow, and kidney beans, along with onions and peppers, are cooked till delicate in a dish. Blend the veggies into the vinegar arrangement and throw to consolidate. Give chill access the refrigerator short-term.

57. Potato Squash Salad

Elements:

- Potatoes, peeled and boiled
- Squash chopped (one cup)
- Flex-meal (one cup)
- Coconut oil (two tbsp)
- Turmeric (half tsp)
- Salt (half tsp)
- Ground cumin (one tbsp)
- Fresh-dill, minced (one tbsp)
- Freshwater (two and a half cups)

Management:

- Hold the SAUTÉ/Heat convention on your Instant pot.

- Set the Coconut-Oil, Brown-Sugar, Vanilla-Extract, and Ground-Cinnamon into the INSTANT POT.

- Continue to form flex-meal and Stir.

- Cook the mixture for four to five minutes.

- Mix it from period to period.

- Next combine water and blend it up.

- Lock the cover and Switch Manual form (High-pressure).

- Add Coconut Oil, Dried Cilantro, Salt, Potatoes, Ground Dark Pepper, Dried Parsley, And Dill.

- Mix the fixings, set Saute mode and cook it for 6-7 minutes.
- Mix time to time.
- At that point add red pepper and white onion. Mix.
- Install the standard mode and warm custard on High for sixteen minutes.
- At that point make fast pressing factor discharge.

Nutrition value:

- Calories (300-307),
- Fat (6.2-7),
- Fiber (5-6),
- Carbs (42.9-43),
- Protein (10-12)

58. Cilantro Brussel Sprouts

Elements:

- Cilantro
- Brussels-sprouts
- Blueberries
- Blackberries
- Coconut milk
- Coconut oil (two tbsp)
- Apples, minced (one cup)
- Freshwater (two and a half cups)
- Brown sugar (two tbsp)
- Vanilla extract (two tbsp)

Management:

- Pour almond milk in the moment pot.
- Combine maple syrup, vanilla concentrate, and sugar. Mix delicately.
- Close the cover and cook on Manual mode (High pressing factor) for five to six minutes.
- At that point make speedy pressing factor discharge.
- Chill the fluid till the room temperature and move in the containers.

- Add cut banana and chia seeds.

- Stir up tenderly.

- Close the container covers and move the pudding in the cooler.

- At that point add coconut yogurt and mix it until homogenous.

- Lock the cover and stay on the yogurt mode for three to four hours.

- At the point when the time is finished – you will get a thick velvety blend.

- Move it on the cheesecloth and press delicately.

- At that point place the yogurt in the yogurt containers.

- Prior to serving add chia seeds, blackberries, and blueberries.

- Formerly perform immediate pressure relief.

- Stir up the meal thoroughly before completing.

- The pudding is cooked in sixty minutes.

Nutrition value:

- Calories (575-580),

- Fat (41.3-41.5),

- Fiber (5-6),

- Carbs (42.9-43),

- Protein (6-8)

Chapter 6

Soups and Stews

59. Tomato-Chicken Soup

Ideal for a chilly autumn day, this soup is hearty and filling. You've got yourself a dinner if you add some bread to it.

Ingredients:

- There should be 6 diced potatoes in there.

- 1 cup The Onion, chopped

- An Ounce and a Half (340 g) Icy corn

- 1 cup low-fat milk

- 14 tsp of garlic powder

- Diced onion, 1 cup (160 g)

- Garlic, minced, 1/2 teaspoon

- There should be 6 diced potatoes in there.

- Carrots, diced, 1 1/2 cups (195 g)

- 1 cup (160 g) (160 g) The Onion, chopped

- 4 cups (950 ml) (950 ml) sodium-reduced chicken stock

- An Ounce and a Half (340 g) Icy corn

- Frozen corn, 10 ounces (280 g)

- Black pepper, half a teaspoon

- Instant mashed potatoes: 1 cup (225 g)

Procedure:

You may soften the potatoes, carrots, and onions by cooking them in stock. Cook some chicken and corn and add it. Just add another 5 minutes of cooking time. Mash the potatoes, then stir in the milk, garlic powder, pepper, and mashed potatoes. The potatoes should be melted completely, so be sure to stir them. Turn up the heat.

60. Soup with Italian Chicken

Here's another dish you can prepare in advance and cook in a slow cooker. This is great to keep on hand for lunches or as a complete supper.

Ingredients:

- Cubed boneless chicken breasts weighing 1 pound (455 g) 4 cups (950 ml) 1 quart (480 g) of low-sodium tomato sauce 2 cups (120 ml) of low-sodium chicken broth

- Diced onion, 1 cup (160 g)

- Garlic, minced, 1/2 tsp

- There should be 6 diced potatoes in there.

- Carrots, diced, half cups (195 g)

- 1 cup The Onion, chopped

- 4 cups sodium-reduced chicken stock

- An Ounce and a Half (340 g) Icy corn

- Frozen corn, 10 ounces (280 g)

- Garlic powder, half a teaspoon

- 1 tsp of dried basil

- The equivalent of one-half teaspoon of oregano

Procedure:

- Put everything in the slow cooker and mix it up. Cook, covered, on low for 8-10 hours or on high for 4-5 hours.

61. Minestrone Soup with Smoked Chicken

This isn't your grandmother's minestrone. The only criteria I had were that it include beans and that it be a good way to finish up the rest of a smoked chicken. Smoked chicken is great, but normal chicken can do in a pinch.

Ingredients:

- Two pieces of smoked chicken thighs

- 2 cups (475 ml) (475 ml) sodium-reduced chicken stock

- Shredded zucchini, 1 cup (113 g)

- Garlic powder, half a teaspoon

- One half cup (50 grams) of chopped celery

- One half cup (65 grams) of sliced carrot

- 1/4 cup (60 g) minced garlic 1 teaspoon (0.4 g) Pâté de chives

- Powdered garlic, equivalent to a quarter teaspoon (0.8 g)

- Two and a half cups (470 ml) of water

- Egg noodles, 12 ounces (340 g)

Procedure:

Rinse the beans once they've been soaked. Chicken should be cooked in a pot with enough stock and water to cover it and simmered until the flesh easily comes off the bones. Remove the meat off the bones and set aside to cool.

It's time to put the meat back in the soup. To cook the beans, add the other ingredients and simmer for 1 1/2 to 2 hours. It may be necessary to add more water. Finish with a sprinkle of Parmesan.

62. Recipe for Amish Chicken Soup

Growing up on the Maryland/Pennsylvania border, Amish chicken corn soup was a staple at the annual carnivals and suppers hosted by the local volunteer fire companies. The soup tastes very much like that one.

Ingredients:

- 4 cups (946 ml) (946 ml) reduced salt chicken broth

- Chicken, cooked and chopped to fill 2 cups (220 g)

- One half cup (50 grams) of chopped celery One half cup (65 grams) of sliced carrot

- 1/4 cup (60 g) minced garlic 1 teaspoon (0.4 g) Pâté de chives

- Powdered garlic, equivalent to a quarter teaspoon (0.8 g)

- Two and a half cups (470 ml) of water

- Egg noodles, 12 ounces (340 g)

- Put everything into a big pot and boil until the noodles are done (by the time indicated on the box).

Procedure:

Chicken may be cooked in water until it's tender. To remove the fat from the soup, chill it. The chicken should be deboned and sliced into bite-sized pieces before being returned to the kettle with the rest of the ingredients.

Put the chicken in a pan and cook it up.

63. Barley and Chicken Soup

Barley makes a welcome departure from the usual chicken noodle or rice soup.

Ingredients:

- Ingredients 2 quarts (1.9 L) water 3 pounds (1.14 kg) of chopped chicken

- 1 1/2 cups (195 g) (195 g) shredded carrots

- 1 cup (120 g) (120 g) shards of celery

- 1 cup (200 g) (200 g) barley with pearls

- 1/2 cup (60 g) (60 g) The Onion, chopped

- Just one bay leaf

- Seasoning for half a teaspoon of chicken

- Black pepper, half a teaspoon

- 12 teaspoon of sage, dried

Procedure:

Chicken may be cooked in water until it's tender. To remove the fat from the soup, chill it. The chicken should be deboned and sliced into bite-sized pieces before being returned to the kettle with the rest of the ingredients.

Put back on the stove and bring to a boil. Cover and simmer for at least an hour, until the veggies are soft and the barley is cooked. Get rid of the bay leaf and dig in.

64. Soup with Chicken, Veggies, and Barley

Flavorful and nutritious, this soup is low in fat and rich in fiber.

Ingredients:

- 4 cups (946 ml) (946 ml) Four cups (720 grams) of low-sodium canned chicken broth

- Water, about 3 cups' worth (710 ml)

- 3 boneless chicken breasts divided into 12 inch (13 mm) cubes, 2 cups (470 ml) reduced salt chicken broth

- Great northern beans, dry; 2 cups (500 grams).

- One Tablespoon (0.7 g) a kind of basil that is normally dried

- Dried oregano, one teaspoon (1 g)

- Can of 2 Cups (360 Grams) Tomatoes without seal

- Cheddar cheese with Parmesan (optional)

- Bay Leaf, One

- Seasoning for 1/2 teaspoon of chicken

- Diced chicken breasts from 2 cups' worth of cooked chicken (around 220 grams)

Procedure:

In a major, weighty pan or Dutch broiler, consolidate everything with the exception of the chicken. The medium intensity ought to be accustomed to heat the blend to the point of boiling. Keep an eye on medium intensity. Stew, blending occasionally, for 45 minutes, or until the vegetables and beans are delicate and the soup is thick. Put the chicken in a skillet and concoct it.

65. Soup with vegetables and Chicken

A comforting bowl of chicken and barley soup on a chilly day.

Ingredients:

- Oil, olive, 2 teaspoons (28 ml)
- Minced celery equaling 1/2 cup (60 g)
- Minced onion, enough to fill 3/4 cup (120 g)
- a level spoonful of flour
- Black pepper, half a teaspoon
- 6 cups (1.4 L) (1.4 L) sodium-reduced chicken stock
- 1 cup (200 g) (200 g) barley with pearls
- 1 pound (455 g) Shredded chicken breasts that were cooked without the bones
- Evaporated skim milk, about a half cup (120 ml)

Procedure:

A hefty pot of oil over medium heat. Mix flour and pepper into the celery and onion before cooking. Incorporate the barley and broth gradually. Flesh out the dish with some chicken. Cook, covered, for an hour or more, stirring regularly, until the barley is soft. Pour in the milk when you remove it from the heat.

66. Chicken Minestrone

A hearty chicken breast stew with all the taste of minestrone.

Ingredients:

- 12 cup (80 g) chopped onion,
- 12 cup (65 g) chopped carrot,
- 1 cup (113 g) diced zucchini, 2 cloves sliced garlic,
- 3 boneless chicken breasts divided into 12 inch
- Great northern beans, dry; 2 cups (500 grams).
- One Tablespoon (0.7 g) a kind of basil that is normally dried
- Dried oregano, one teaspoon (1 g)
- Can of 2 Cups (360 Grams) Tomatoes without seal
- Cheddar cheese with Parmesan (optional)

Procedure:

Sauté the vegetables (onion, carrot, zucchini, and garlic) until soft. Blend with the rest of the soup's elements and simmer for a further hour and a half. If more liquid is required, add it now. If you like, sprinkle some Parmesan cheese on top.

67. African a Stew made with Peanuts

Spicy peanut-flavored vegetable stew with sweet potatoes and other veggies.

Ingredients:

- One turkey carcass, with the majority of the flesh trimmed off
- 2.8 liters (3 quarts) of water
- one table spoon of peppercorns
- Celery, diced, one cup (100 g)
- Onion, chopped, 2 cups (320 g)
- Chicken broth, around 4 cups (950 ml)
- Dry red wine, one cup (around 235 ml)
- 1 1/2 cups finely diced onion
- The equivalent of 2 cups (300 grams) of chopped turnip.
- 2 cups (470 ml) Salinity-reduced tomato juice
- peanut butter, low-fat, 1/2 cup (130 g)

Procedure:

- Cut a yam into shapes and cook it in water until it's delicate. Get some oil hot in a major cooker over medium intensity. Cook the garlic, ginger, coriander, and cayenne powder briefly in a sauté container. Put in certain onions and stew them down until they're delicate. Stew the tomato-eggplant combination for ten minutes subsequent to adding the water. Throw in the zucchini and pepper and continue to cook at a low stew for an additional 20 minutes, or until everything is delicate. Stuff yams, tomato fluid, and peanut butter into a stew. Yams ought to be cooked in something like 15 minutes in the event that they are stewed over low intensity with steady blending.

68. Soup Made from a Turkey's Remains

This is a special and nutritious process to use the any leftover turkey from Thanksgiving.

Ingredients:

- One turkey carcass, with the majority of the flesh trimmed off
- 2.8 liters (3 quarts) of water
- one table spoon of peppercorns
- Celery, diced, one cup (100 g)
- Onion, chopped, 2 cups (320 g)

- Chicken broth, around 4 cups (950 ml)

- Dry red wine, one cup (around 235 ml)

- 1 1/2 cups finely diced onion

- The equivalent of 2 cups (300 grams) of chopped turnip.

Procedure:

Water should just reach the top of the turkey carcass in a big saucepan. Spice it up with some pepper and some chopped onion and celery. For 45 minutes, let it simmer. Recover any residual meat from the corpse after draining and saving the fluids. Simmer the beef for 30 minutes in the liquid you preserved, along with some chicken stock and red wine. Put in the remaining components. Soak rice and barley for at least 45 minutes and up to 2 hours, depending on their size.

69. Meat soup

Barley makes for an interesting alternative to the usual chicken noodle or rice soup.

Ingredients:

- 2 quarts (1.9 L) water 3 pounds (1.14 kg) of chicken breasts

- 1 1/2 cups (195 g) Cut Carrots

- 1 cup (120 g) chop celery

- 1 cup (200 g) little grains of wheat

- 1/2 cup (60 g) onions, chopped

- Bay Leaf, One

- Seasoning for 1/2 teaspoon of chicken

- 1/2 milligram of pepper

- 12 tsp of ground sage

Procedure:

- Heat chicken to the point of boiling, then, at that point, decrease intensity and stew until cooked through. Set the stock's temperature to cool and eliminate the fat. Eliminate chicken from bones and cleave into reduced down pieces, then add back to the bubble alongside the other fixings.

- Return to the oven and bring the temperature up to boiling again. Cover and cook over low intensity, blending at times, for essentially more than one hour, or the veggies are smooth and the grain is baked. Simply take out the narrows leaf and serve.

- Roughly 6 servings might be gotten from this recipe.

70. Vegetable Chicken Barley Soup

This healthy soup has a lot of flavors, is low in fat, and is rich in fiber.

Ingredients:

- 4 cups (946 ml) (946 ml) Four cups (720 grams) of low-sodium chicken broth in a can Tomatoes without additional salt

- There should be three cups (710 ml) of water.

- 1/4 cup (50 g) (50 g) little grains of wheat

- Split peas, about a quarter cup (50 grams)

- 1.5 tablespoons (3 g) Sage leaves that have been dried

- Diced cooked chicken breasts to fill 2 cups (220 grams)

Procedure:

- Put everything with the exception of the chicken into a major, weighty pot like a Dutch stove and blend well. Begin a bubble utilizing a medium intensity source.

- Decrease the intensity to medium. Soup ought to be thick and vegetables and vegetables delicate following 45 minutes of stewing, during which time they ought to be blended occasionally. Then, place the chicken in the container and simmer until done.

71. Bowl of Chicken Barley Chowder

A hearty chicken and barley soup that is both easy to make and satisfying on a chilly day.

Ingredients:

- Olive oil, enough for 2 teaspoons (28 ml)
- Celery, minced, about a half cup (60 g)
- 120 g (three-quarters of a cup) of chopped onion
- One Tablespoon of Flour
- 1/2 milligram of pepper
- Dry red wine, one cup (around 235 ml)
- 1 1/2 cups finely diced onion
- The equivalent of 2 cups (300 grams) of chopped turnip.
- One-third of a cup of rice (97 grams)
- 1/2 cup (100 g) (100 g) little grains of wheat
- Fat-free evaporated milk, about a half cup (120 ml)

Procedure:

- Warm the oil in the huge pot. Flour and pepper might be added to the celery and onion that has been sautéed.

- Add the broth and grain to the pot gradually, and blend well.

- Consolidate some chicken. Keep covered and stew for 60 minutes, blending intermittently, until grain is delicate. Remove the intensity and pour in some milk.

72. Chicken breast pieces

Minestrone with diced chicken breast is a hearty dish that adds a meaty texture and savory taste.

Ingredients:

- Dry red wine, one cup (around 235 ml)
- 1 1/2 cups finely diced onion
- The equivalent of 2 cups (300 grams) of chopped turnip.
- One-third of a cup of rice (97 grams)
- 1/2 cup (100 g) (100 g) little grains of wheat
- Dry Great Northern Beans, 2 cups (500 grams)
- Size: 1 tsp (0.7 g) Basil leaves, dried
- Dry Oregano, One Gram, One Tablespoon
- 2 cups (360 g) of canned Tomatoes without additional salt
- Grass-fed, aged Parmesan (optional)

Procedure:

- Put a few onions, carrots, zucchini, and garlic in a container and cook them until they're delicate.

- Join with the other soup's fixings in a huge pan and bubble for 1 1/2 hours.

- Assuming more fluid is required, feel free to add it. Parmesan cheddar might be utilized as an enhancement.

73. African Stewed Peanuts

A peanut-butter-flavored, spicy vegetarian stew that features sweet potatoes and other veggies.

Ingredients:

- 2 teaspoons of oil 2 tablespoons of diced sweet potato (30 ml) Oil from canola seeds
- a half teaspoon of minced garlic (1.5 g)
- 1 inch of fresh ginger, minced
- Ground coriander: 2 teaspoons (12 g)
- 12 tsp. (0.9 g) cayenne pepper

Procedure:

- To cook yam 3D shapes, you may either steam them or bubble them. To begin, heat the oil in a large pan over medium heat. For 1 moment, bake oil in a skillet and add garlic, ginger, coriander, and cayenne pepper. Put in the onions, and cook them down until they're delicate. Blend in the tomatoes, eggplant, and water, and heat at a low stew for 10 minutes.

• At the point when the eggplant and potatoes are cooked, add the zucchini and ringer pepper and keep stewing for an additional 20 minutes. Put a few yams in the stew alongside some peanut butter and tomato juice. Stew over low intensity, mixing periodically, for 15 minutes, or until yams are delicate.

74. Bowl of Turkey Bone Broth

The best way to use up any leftover turkey from Thanksgiving; tasty and nutritious.

Ingredients:

• One turkey carcass, with most of the flesh gone

• Just under 3 liters (1 quart)

• Peppercorns, one tablespoon's worth

• 100 grams (one cup) of chopped celery

• Approximately 2 cups (320 grams) of finely chopped onion

• (4 x 950 ml) cups of chicken broth

• Dry red wine, one cup (around 235 ml)

• 1 1/2 cups finely diced onion

• The equivalent of 2 cups (300 grams) of chopped turnip.

• One-third of a cup of rice (97 grams)

• 1/2 cup (100 g) (100 g) little grains of wheat

Procedure:

• Put turkey body in a significant pot and add scarcely adequate water to cover it. Consolidate the peppercorns and a big part of the cleaved onion and celery.

• Cook at a low stew for 45 minutes. Now is the ideal time to deplete the remains, save the juices for sometime in the future, and look over it for any leftover tissue.

• Consolidate the meat, stock, and wine that was saved, and bubble for 30 minutes. Throw in the leftover parts. Keep stewing for no less than 45 minutes and as long as 2 hours, or until rice and grain are delicate.

Chapter 7

Fish and Seafood

75. Salmon fillets on the grill

For this dish, a complete salmon fillet would do just fine. Even though it's a bit of a pain to maneuver, the spectacle it puts up is well worth the effort. Typically, I'll chop the fillet into manageable halves, but you still need to be cautious not to overcook it and make it tough. Salmon is complemented by the sauce's mild sweetness.

Ingredients:

- 1/4 cup sugar, brown

- Apple cider vinegar, 2 teaspoons (or 30 ml)

- 30 milliliters (2 teaspoons) of honey

- One milliliter (or a quarter teaspoon) of liquid smoke

- Pepper, black, one-fourth teaspoon (0.5 g)

- About a quarter of a teaspoon (0.8 g) minced or crushed garlic

Procedure:

- Ready the grill. The first six ingredients (through garlic) should be mixed together in a small basin. Don't be stingy with the mixing. Apply the basting sauce to one side of the salmon, then set it on the grill with the sauced side facing down. Halfway through grilling, baste the salmon's top side and turn the fillet so the new basting sauce is now facing the heat. Apply the basting sauce and turn the salmon one more when the cooking time is almost up. Finish the salmon by basting it and flipping it over before serving.

76. Salmon with Cedar Planks

Salmon prepared on a wood board while grilling takes on a fantastic smokey taste. Grilling it without any sauce is OK, however we recommend this honey mustard sauce.

Ingredients:

- 1/4 cup (60 g) (60 g) A condiment known as Dijon
- Honey, 1 tablespoon (15 ml)
- Dried dill, one teaspoon (1 g)
- salmon fillets weighing 1 pound (455 g)

Procedure:

In a bowl, combine the mustard, honey, and dill. Use to marinade salmon in a glass baking dish before throwing it on the grill. Prepare the grill by preheating it to medium and soaking the planks as directed on the packaging. To warm a plank, just place it on a preheated grill for three minutes. Salmon goes on the board after it has been flipped over. Grill lid must be in place for the whole 12 minutes for the fish to flake easily.

77. Salmon roasted with thyme

Even though there are just three ingredients in this dish, the salmon is packed with flavor.

Ingredients:

• Fillets of fish weighing 1 pound

• The equivalent of one teaspoon of dried thyme

• Black pepper, one-fourth teaspoon

Procedure:

• Prepare a baking sheet by spraying it with nonstick spray. Set the fillets on the sheet.

• Season with thyme and pepper. Fish will be ready after 20 minutes in the oven at 350 degrees Fahrenheit.

78. Salmon with Honey Mustard Glaze

Salmon already has a little sweetness, so the honey mustard glaze works well.

Ingredients:

• Fillets of fish weighing 1 pound

• honey, 2 tbsp

• 1 teaspoon of ground mustard

• A pinch of thyme

• olive oil, 1 table spoon

Procedure:

• In a big, nonstick pan, heat the oil over medium heat. Blend together the honey, mustard, and thyme. To prepare the fish, brush all sides. Fish should be fried for approximately 5 minutes each side in oil until it flakes easily.

79. Atlantic Salmon from the Mediterranean

Not only does this whole dinner look beautiful, but it also tastes fantastic.

Ingredients:

- salmon fillets weighing 1 pound (455 g)

- Couscous, one cup (175 g)

- A cup of zucchini (113 g), sliced

- red onion (160 g),

- mushrooms (sliced)

- honey, 2 tbsp

- 1 teaspoon of ground mustard

- A pinch of thyme

- olive oil, 1 table spoon

- (2 tbsp / 30 ml) of olive oil, measured out

- basil, fresh, 1 tbsp (2.5 g)

Procedure:

- Follow the directions on the couscous packet to make it. For the time being, heat up a frying pan or griddle. Stir the oil into the zucchini, onion, mushrooms, and red bell pepper. The veggies should be sautéed for 8-10 minutes, turned once.

- Take out of the oven. Toss the salmon with the last tablespoon of oil (15 ml) and fry for 6-8 minutes, rotating once. Toss the couscous with the veggies and basil. Accompany the salmon with a serving of veggie couscous.

80. Salmon with Vegetables Baked in the Oven

I have also used a gas grill to prepare this.

Ingredients:

- fillets of salmon weighing 8 ounces (225 grams)

- 2 diced medium potatoes

- honey, 2 tbsp

- 1 teaspoon of ground mustard

- A pinch of thyme

- olive oil, 1 table spoon

Procedure:

• Set oven temperature to 425F (220C), or gas mark 7. Make sure to also preheat a baking sheet. Spray the middle of two pieces of 12-by-12-by-30-centimeter aluminum foil with nonstick vegetable oil spray.

• Prepare several sheets of foil and distribute the salmon, potatoes, squash, carrots, onions, and mushrooms among them. Wine, dill, garlic, and pepper are sprinkled over a square of dough before it is folded diagonally to make a triangle and the corners are sealed.

• Return the baking sheet to the oven and bake for another 10–15 minutes, or until the salmon is opaque and the veggies are soft if cooked separately.

81. Tuna Steaks

Tuna steaks are high in healthy omega-3 fatty acids and, if purchased on sale, may be very cost-effective. To avoid drying them out, avoid cooking them for too long. You may enjoy them quite well cooked at the medium or even medium-rare temperature. A simple marinade may be used to keep them juicy and flavored as they cook.

Ingredients:

• 30 milliliters (2 tablespoons) of olive oil

• Juice from 2 lemons, around 30 milliliters

• Tuna steaks, six ounces (170 grams)

• Black pepper, freshly ground, half a teaspoon (1 gram)

Procedure:

Olive oil and lemon juice should be mixed together. Marinate the steaks for 30 minutes, flipping them over halfway through. A pan or skillet should be heated at high heat. You just need two minutes to cook the steaks after adding them. Toss in some pepper, flip, and cook for another two minutes.

82. Steaks of Tuna in a Delicious Marinade

The southwestern marinade on these tuna steaks pairs well with the Spanish rice and maize.

Ingredients:

• Two Tablespoons (about 30 mL) of Olive Oil

• 2 tsp. (5 g) (5 g) cumin

• 2 tbsp of fresh lime juice (or 30 ml)

• Chopped cilantro, 2 teaspoons (2.6 grams)

• One-pound tuna steaks (455 grams)

Procedure:

•   Combine the first four ingredients in a pie plate or other shallow dish, then add the fish and turn to coat. After preparing the marinade, let the meat marinate in it for 20 minutes, turning once halfway through. Fire up the grill to a high temperature. Remove the tuna from the marinade and sear it over high heat for two minutes on each side.

83. Sashimi-Style Poached Salmon

Poaching is a great way to prepare fish because it retains the food's natural flavor and moisture without adding too much oil.

Ingredients:

•   four glasses' worth of water (946 ml)

•   two lemons' worth of juice, or 30 ml

•   Approximately one-fourth cup of finely sliced carrots (30 g)

•   1/2 cup of finely chopped onion (80 g)

•   Exceptional Bay Leaf, Top Pick

•   fresh dill, about 1/2 pound, diced Salmon fillets, 1 tablespoon (4 g) (225 g

Procedure:

•   Crank up the oven temperature to 350 degrees Fahrenheit (180 degrees Celsius, or gas mark 4). Bring everything to a boil except the fish. Allow to cook slowly for 5 minutes.

•   Pour the poaching liquid into a glass baking dish that is large enough to hold a single layer of salmon. After 20 minutes in the oven, the salmon, if covered, should be flaky.

84. Salmon fillets

Salmon complements the balsamic vinegar and maple syrup's complementary sweet and savory flavors.

Ingredients:

•   Vinegar, balsamic, 1/4 cup (60 ml)

•   The equivalent of one-fourth of a cup of water (60 ml)

•   30 milliliters (2 tablespoons) of olive oil

•   Add 2 tbsp (30 ml) Sweetener: Maple Syrup

•   a garlic powder equivalent to a quarter teaspoon (0.8 g)

•   225 grams (half a pound) of salmon fillets

Procedure:

• Salmon is optional. Heat all ingredients except salmon in a large pan, stirring often. Prepare salmon fillets and include them. Ten minutes, covered, flipping once, will get you well cooked fish.

85. The Salmon and Veggies Are Grilled

In extreme heat, it may be best to avoid using the stove at all. In this meal, protein, veggies, and grains are all grilled together for convenience.

Ingredients:

• Uncooked instant rice, one cup (195 g)

• 1 cup broth made with minimal levels of salt from chicken

• a quarter of a zucchini (56 g) sliced

• Carrot, shredded, about a half cup (60 g)

• 225 grams (half a pound) of salmon fillets

• Pepper, black, one-fourth teaspoon (0.5 g)

• The juice of half a lemon

Procedure:

• Grill to medium heat. Nonstick vegetable oil spray on two huge sheets of heavy-duty aluminum foil. The rice and broth should be combined in a separate dish. The broth should be allowed to sit for 5 minutes. Add the zucchini and carrots and put aside. Place a salmon fillet in the center of each aluminum foil sheet.

• Add pepper and lemon slices for garnish. Wrap the fillets in the rice mixture. Align the foil's edges and fold it in half. Seal by folding over multiple times to create a tight fold.

• Leave a little gap at the ends for the rice to expand during cooking. Ten to fifteen minutes on the grill should be enough time to cook the salmon.

86. Mediterranean Tilapia

These otherwise unassuming fillets are topped with a delicious mixture of sun-dried tomatoes and olives, which adds a wonderful depth of flavor.

Ingredients:

• 8 pitted, chopped olives 1/4 cup chopped sun-dried tomatoes in oil 2 tablespoons diced pimento

• Parsley, fresh, 2 tablespoons

• Basil, fresh, 1 tbsp

- olive oil, 1 table spoon

- Four fillets of tilapia

- A Pinch of Paprika

- Cayenne Pepper, 1/8 Teaspoon

Procedure:

- Prepare a baking sheet by spraying it with nonstick spray. Blend together the tomatoes, olives, pimiento, parsley, basil, and oil. Putting aside. Arrange fillets in baking dish. Cayenne pepper and paprika may be sprinkled on top. To cook fish in the oven, set the temperature to 400 degrees Fahrenheit and wait around 15 minutes. Place on plates and cover with the tomato sauce.

87. Islands of Greece Fish

Enjoying this fish will make you feel like you've teleported to a tropical paradise in the Mediterranean. Accompany couscous.

Ingredients:

- 6 fillets of tilapia

- Diced tomatoes (no salt added) to equal 1 cup

- 1/4 cup chopped spinach

- 12 cup chopped olives, preferably ripe

- crumbled feta cheese equaling 1/2 cup

Procedure:

- Coat a 9-by-13-inch baking sheet with nonstick cooking spray and add the fillets. Sprinkle with the rest of the ingredients. Fish should flake readily when baked for 15–20 minutes at 400°F.

88. Baked Tuna

This dish epitomizes the concept of American comfort food.

Ingredients:

- The equivalent of one tablespoon (15 ml) of olive oil

- 2 cups (470 ml) milk that has been diluted to a skim

- Any solid white fish weighing 2 pounds (905 g), such as perch

- 1/2 teaspoon (15 ml) oil of olive

- 1/2 milliliter (1.5 g) The Communal Garlic Herb and Spice Blend

- 1/2 milliliter (0.3 g) marjoram, dried

- 1/2 milliliter (0.5 g) thyme, dried

- white pepper, 1/8 teaspoon (0.3 g)

Procedure:

- To heat effectively, get your broiler up to 375 degrees Fahrenheit (190 degrees Celsius, or gas mark 5). Oil ought to be warmed over low intensity in a major dish prior to adding flour and mixing continually until a smooth glue structures. Mixing constantly, cook for 1 moment.

- Add the milk steadily and stew, blending every now and again, until the sauce has thickened and is gurgling. Toss in the cheddar and continue to throw while you cook it over low intensity to guarantee it softens. Take it off the oven at this moment.

89. Fish with Herbs

Herbs and spices provide depth of flavor to otherwise bland baked fish.

Ingredients:

- any solid white fish weighing 2 pounds (905 g), such as perch

- 1/2 teaspoon (15 ml) oil of olive

- 1/2 milliliter (1.5 g) The Communal Garlic Herb and Spice Blend

- 1/2 milliliter (0.3 g) marjoram, dried

- 1/2 milliliter (0.5 g) thyme, dried

- white pepper, 1/8 teaspoon (0.3 g)

- (Two) Bay Leaves

Procedure:

Turn the oven temperature up to 350 degrees Fahrenheit (180 degrees Celsius, or gas mark 4). Fish should be washed and dried before being placed in a 9 by 13-inch (23 by 33-cm) dish. Garlic powder, marjoram, thyme, and white pepper may be added to oil. Squeeze over fish. Sprinkle some onion and bay leaves over top. A glass of wine should be poured over everything. If you want flaky fish, check it after 20 to 30 minutes of baking in an uncovered dish.

90. Pan-Fried Fish

The low-fat and low-sodium coating is perfect for pairing with oven-fried potatoes, and the crunch is a welcome addition.

Ingredients:

- 1 egg

- Add 2 tbsp (30 ml) milk that has been diluted to a skim

- Dry potato flakes, about 1/2 cup (30 g)

- About a quarter of a teaspoon (0.5 g) A spice called black pepper

- 1 pound (455 g) fillets of catfish

Procedure:

Set oven temperature to 325F (170C/gas 3) and get it hot. Blend the egg with the milk. Potatoes and pepper should be mixed together. Coat fish with the egg and potato mixture, and then coat it in flakes. Soak the fish in egg once more, and then coat it with potato flakes. Arrange on a pan for baking. Spray vegetable oil spray that doesn't stay on fish. Fish should flake readily after 15 minutes in the oven.

91. Recipe for Tuna and Brown Rice Bake

Similar to a tuna casserole, but with a few twists. Brown rice boosts the meal's nutritional value, while yogurt adds both taste and smoothness.

- 1 Raw brown rice, about a quarter cup (238 g)

- Water, around three cups' worth (or 710 ml)

- One hundred grams (one cup) of chopped celery

- Onion, finely diced, 1/2 cup (80 g)

- 1/2 cup (115 g) (115 g) Yogurt, fat-free and plain

- 1 cup (235 ml) (235 ml) milk that has been diluted to a skim

- Red pepper flakes, about a quarter teaspoon (0.3 g)

Procedure:

- Turn the broiler temperature up to 350 degrees Fahrenheit (180 degrees Celsius, or gas mark 4). A major pot is ideal for joining the rice and water. Raise the temperature until a bubble structures. Cover and cook on low intensity for 35 minutes. Take it off the oven at the present time.

- Mix in the tarragon, tarragon, red pepper pieces, celery, onion, yogurt, milk, and red onion. After the rice has cooled, add the frozen peas and chipped fish and mix to join. Add to a goulash dish that holds 2 quarts (1.9 liters). Put it in the broiler for 30 minutes. Spread some destroyed cheddar on top.

92. Tuna Casserole

Have you ever been at a loss for what to make for supper and found yourself rummaging aimlessly through cookbooks in search of a recipe that sounded nice and used materials you already had on hand? The end outcome was this. Moreover, the outcome was positive. An eggy custard, reminiscent of quiche, forms the top layer.

Ingredients:

- Cooked rice, 2 cups (330 g)

- Four eggs, each apportioned to a quarter of a teaspoon (0.7 g) Basil, Dried

- One tenth of a cup (10 g) of chopped onion

- 200 grams (7 ounces) of water pre-prepared tuna

- 1 cup (235 ml) (235 ml) milk that has been diluted to a skim

- A measure of 4 ounces (115 g) crumbled Swiss cheese

Procedure:

Turn the broiler temperature up to 350 degrees Fahrenheit (180 degrees Celsius, or gas mark 4). Blended 1 egg, rice, basil, and onion. Put the blend into a nonstick 8-by-8-inch (20-by-20-cm) baking dish. Put some fish on top. Pour the excess milk, cheddar, and egg blend on top. A blade embedded towards the center ought to tell the truth following 40 to 45 minutes of baking.

93. Baked Tuna and Noodles

This dish epitomizes the concept of American comfort food.

Ingredients:

- The equivalent of one tablespoon (15 ml) of olive oil

- 2 cups (470 ml) milk that has been diluted to a skim

- Any solid white fish weighing 2 pounds (905 g), such as perch

- 1/2 teaspoon (15 ml) oil of olive

- 1/2 milliliter (1.5 g) The Communal Garlic Herb and Spice Blend

- 1/2 milliliter (0.3 g) marjoram, dried

- 1/2 milliliter (0.5 g) thyme, dried

- white pepper, 1/8 teaspoon (0.3 g)

Procedure:

• To heat effectively, get your broiler up to 375 degrees Fahrenheit (190 degrees Celsius, or gas mark 5). Oil ought to be warmed over low intensity in a major dish prior to adding flour and mixing continually until a smooth glue structures. Mixing constantly, cook for 1 moment.

• Add the milk steadily and stew, blending every now and again, until the sauce has thickened and is gurgling. Toss in the cheddar and continue to throw while you cook it over low intensity to guarantee it softens. Take it off the oven at this moment.

94. Fish with Herbs

Herbs and spices provide depth of flavor to otherwise bland baked fish.

• any solid white fish weighing 2 pounds (905 g), such as perch

• 1/2 teaspoon (15 ml) oil of olive

• 1/2 milliliter (1.5 g) The Communal Garlic Herb and Spice Blend

• 1/2 milliliter (0.3 g) marjoram, dried

• 1/2 milliliter (0.5 g) thyme, dried

• white pepper, 1/8 teaspoon (0.3 g)

• (Two) Bay Leaves

Procedure:

Turn the oven temperature up to 350 degrees Fahrenheit (180 degrees Celsius, or gas mark 4). Fish should be washed and dried before being placed in a 9 by 13-inch (23 by 33-cm) dish. Garlic powder, marjoram, thyme, and white pepper may be added to oil. Squeeze over fish. Sprinkle some onion and bay leaves over top. A glass of wine should be poured over everything. If you want flaky fish, check it after 20 to 30 minutes of baking in an uncovered dish.

95. Pan-Fried Fish

The low-fat and low-sodium coating is perfect for pairing with oven-fried potatoes, and the crunch is a welcome addition.

Ingredients:

• 1 egg

• Add 2 tbsp (30 ml) milk that has been diluted to a skim

• Dry potato flakes, about 1/2 cup (30 g)

• About a quarter of a teaspoon (0.5 g) A spice called black pepper

• 1 pound (455 g) fillets of catfish

Procedure:

Set oven temperature to 325F (170C/gas 3) and get it hot. Blend the egg with the milk. Potatoes and pepper should be mixed together. Coat fish with the egg and potato mixture, and then coat it in flakes. Soak the fish in egg once more, and then coat it with potato flakes. Arrange on a pan for baking. Spray vegetable oil spray that doesn't stay on fish. Fish should flake readily after 15 minutes in the oven.

96. Pan-Fried Catfish with Pecans

A tasty southern delicacy. Pair with a pilaf of rice.

Ingredients:

- Dijon mustard, 6 teaspoons (90 g)

- The equivalent of one-fourth of a cup (60 ml) of low-fat milk

- Amount: 1 cup (100 g) ground pecans

- catfish fillets weighing 1 pound (455 g)

Procedure:

Set oven temperature to 450F (230C, gas mark 8). Use a vegetable oil-free cooking spray to coat a baking sheet. Place the mustard and milk in a small bowl and mix together. Nuts, in another dish, were spread out. Coat fillets with a mustard and honey mixture, then roll them in pecans. Put on the baking sheet you just made. Bake until salmon flakes easily, about 10 to 12 minutes.

97. The Catfish is Baked

This bread crumb-topped catfish is simple to prepare and pairs well with any meal.

Ingredients:

- Fish fillets weighing one pound

- Seasoning for Italian cooking, half a teaspoon

- 1/4 cup soft bread crumbs

- 1 stick of melted unsalted butter

Procedure:

- To bake well, an oven temperature of 425 degrees Fahrenheit must be maintained. Spray nonstick cooking spray onto baking dish. Season the fish with Italian seasoning and bread crumbs, then place it in a skillet. Put a little bit of melted butter on top. It takes around 20 minutes in the oven until the fish is flaky.

98. Salmon Patties

Growing older, canned salmon was more affordable than tuna. Salmon patties were a staple in our house since they were both easy to prepare and delicious. Even though salmon isn't as cheap as it once was, these patties are delicious.

Ingredients:

- Drained and flaked salmon from a 14-ounce (400-g) can

- 2 eggs

- Olive oil, one tablespoon (around 15 ml)

- Shallots, minced (1 tablespoon)

- 1/2 milligram of garlic powder

- a heaping tablespoon of chopped fresh parsley

- Fresh basil, minced, 2 teaspoons

Procedure:

- Blend the salmon, eggs, bread scraps, onion, salt, and pepper in a huge bowl, then, at that point, partition the combination into six equivalent divides and structure into patties.

- A major griddle with oil in it ought to be warmed over medium intensity. Put in the salmon cakes and cook until brilliant.

99. A Scallop-Topped Linguine Dish

It always feels like a celebration when seafood is on the menu. Scallops elevate an otherwise standard spaghetti dish to gourmet status.

Ingredients:

- Olive oil, one tablespoon (around 15 ml)

- Shallots, minced (1 tablespoon)

- 1/2 milligram of garlic powder

- a heaping tablespoon of chopped fresh parsley

- Fresh basil, minced, 2 teaspoons

- 455 grams, or about 1 pound, of scallops

- Artichoke hearts, thawed (9 oz/255 g)

Procedure:

- Cooking oil ought to be warmed over medium intensity in a 3-quart (3-L) pot. Consolidate the garlic and shallots and cook for an additional 3 minutes. Throw in certain spices and flavors like parsley, basil, pepper drops, tomatoes, wine, and tomato glue. Tomatoes ought to be separated while they bubble in the pot. Set the clock for 20 minutes and cover the pot.

• Slice colossal scallops down the middle the long way. Blend in the scallops and artichoke hearts with the tomatoes. Scallops and artichokes need about 5 minutes in the stove to get their ideal doneness.

• Linguine ought to be ready as per bundle headings, then depleted. Spread pasta on a serving plate and top with the scallop blend, then, at that point, sprinkle with pine nuts. Adding a basil leaf as an enhancement is discretionary.

100. Fish and Spaghetti

Inspiring by a similar dish she saw on a cooking show, my daughter prepared this. It was a success, and it's just different enough from how we usually serve pasta that we go back to it when we want something a bit different; anyway, it follows my daughter's rule that if you don't know what to have, create something Italian.

Ingredients:

• Spaghetti, about 8 ounces (225 grams)

• white fish, such as perch, weighing 1 pound (455 g)

• (2 Tablespoons) (30 ml) We use olive oil when we cook.

• 1/2 milliliter (1.5 g) garlic, minced

• (2 Tablespoons) (30 ml) Concentrated lemon extract

• 1/2 teaspoon (2.5 g) Spices from Italy

• Exactly one-fourth of a teaspoon (0.5 g) cracked black pepper

• 2 cups (360 g) (360 g) canned salt-free tomato sauce

• 1/4 cup (60 ml) (60 ml) Sauvignon Blanc

Procedure:

• It is prescribed to get ready pasta as per bundle rules, barring the utilization of salt. Put away some the pasta cooking water. Throw the cooked pasta.

• Set up a medium intensity in a major skillet. Acquire the wine and the shrimp. Close the cover and stew for 1-2 minutes, or until the shrimp become pink and misty.

101. Pasta with Tuna Sauce

Instead of scallops, tuna can be used to make a fancy Italian dish.

Ingredients:

- A total of 3/4 cup (175 ml) olive oil, divided
- 1 cup bell pepper, green, sliced
- Sliced red bell pepper, 1 cup (150 g)
- 1 cup prepared with chopped yellow bell pepper
- The mushrooms were cut and added.
- 1 cup -thin rings of onion
- One teaspoon of minced garlic
- White tuna, one can
- 3/4 cup (175 ml) (175 ml) white wine that's dry
- Only 4 ounces (115 g) grated romano cheese

Procedure:

Bring the pan up to temperature. 1/4 cup of olive oil should be enough to cover the bottom of the pan. Put in some garlic, onions, mushrooms, and peppers. Cook in a pan till tender but still somewhat crunchy. Pour in the remaining oil. Blend in the wine and tuna. Stir. Mix in some parsley and cheese. Stack it on top of linguine that's been prepared per the package's instructions.

102. Tuna Tacos

Are you in need of a fast meal for lunch or dinner? These tacos need no cooking and are both flavorful and nutritious.

Ingredients:

- 6 1 and a half ounces (184 g) of tuna, deboned and flakes
- 1/3 cup (33 g) (33 g) scallion pieces
- One-fourth of a cup (or 65 grams) of salsa
- 2 cups (110 g) (110 g) lettuce that has been shredded
- Eight corn tortillas
- Drain and rinse 1 cup (164 grams) chickpeas
- Tomatoes, chopped: 1 cup (180 g)

- ripe olives, a scant 1/3 cup (33 g)

Procedure:

Mix tuna, scallions, and salsa in a medium bowl. Putting together tacos entails: Distribute some lettuce among the taco fillings. Evenly distribute the tuna mixture, chickpeas, tomatoes, and olives among the tacos. Add condiments to taste.

103. Sesame Fish

Crunchy and flavorful sesame seeds top off this Asian-inspired baked fish.

Ingredients:

- 1 pound (455 g) canned halibut fillets
- 1/2 cup (120 ml) (120 ml) Teriyaki sauce with less salt, like Dick's (recipe on page 25).
- (2 Tablespoons) (16 g) The seeds of the sesame plant
- 8 grams flour may be divided into 1 tablespoon.
- one gram of white pepper (half a teaspoon)

Procedure:

- Filets ought to be organized in a solitary layer in a shallow baking dish. Fish with teriyaki sauce. Put in the cooler for somewhere around 30 minutes, ideally short-term. Set up a 450F (230C) stove (gas mark 8). Blend some flour, pepper, and sesame seeds together.

- Eggs and milk ought to be combined as one in a little bowl. Put some pepper on it. Shower a pie dish with nonstick vegetable oil splash, then, at that point, spread portion of the cheddar in the base. Spread the cheddar first, then the onions, then get done with the tomatoes. Sprinkle the veggies with the egg combination.

- Season with the excess cheddar and serve. Put it in the broiler and set the clock for 10 minutes. Prepare for 15-20 minutes, or until filling is puffed and brilliant brown, at a decreased intensity of 350°F (180°C or gas mark 4). Serve hot.

104. Salad with Tuna and Pasta

When the weather is hot and you don't feel like cooking, this salad may serve as your main course.

Ingredients:

- Weighing in at a mere 8 ounces (225 g) Spaghetti made with 100% whole wheat
- 1/2 pound (225 g) green pods of a pea plant
- There is just enough tuna for one can.
- Size: 6 oz (170 g) Hearts of artichoke
- a half a cup of sliced green olives (around 50 grams)
- 35 grams (1/2 pound) of freshly sliced mushrooms
- 1/2 cup (120 ml) (120 ml) Dressing, Italian

81

- 1/3 of a teaspoon of lemon pepper
- Grated Parmesan cheese, about a quarter cup (25 g)

Procedure:

Pasta should be cooked to package guidelines, then drained and allowed to cool. Pea pods need just a minute in boiling water before they are ready to be removed and set aside to cool. Gather the empty pods and shells in a container. Tuna, after being rinsed, may be added to a dish of pea pods. Include mushrooms, olives, artichoke hearts, and artichoke juice. Toss with spaghetti and dress with the dressing. Toss in some ground lemon pepper and stir to combine. Put some Parmesan on top.

105. Salad with Tuna, White Beans, and Pasta

One serving of this delicious main course salad provides about half of the recommended daily fiber intake.

Ingredients:

- Vegetables
- Artichoke hearts, one can
- 6 ounces of green beans (170 grams), blanched and drained
- beets, half a pound (225 g), cooked or canned, drained, and sliced
- Tomatoes, cut into wedges (1 1/2 cups/270 g)
- Pasta Mixture
- 225 grams (1/2 pound) of cooked, drained, and washed whole wheat pasta
- 2 cups (200 grams) of cooked, drained white beans
- 1 drained can of tuna
- Vinaigrette
- 60 ml (1/4 cup) of olive oil
- 1/2 cup (120 ml) (120 ml) Lemon juice that has just been squeezed from a lemon
- Minced garlic (one half of a clove)
- 1/2 fresh basil leaf
- Black pepper, half a teaspoon

Procedure:

Mix the vinaigrette ingredients together using a whisk. Marinate the veggies for at least an hour in half of the vinaigrette mixture. Combine the pasta, beans, and tuna in a single bowl once they have been drained. Combine the remaining vinaigrette with the vegetable-pasta combination just before serving.

106. Pasta with Shrimp and Spinach

Flavor is subtle, but you can't go wrong with the health benefits and deliciousness of shrimp and spinach.

Ingredients:

- Whole wheat pasta, 6 ounces

- 1 lb. peeled shrimp

- Two-thirds of a cup of white wine, dry

- Approximately 2 teaspoons of olive oil

- 1 cup of sliced onion

- a minced clove of garlic equaling one teaspoon

- One kilogram of fresh spinach

Procedure:

- It is prescribed to get ready pasta as per bundle rules, barring the utilization of salt. Put away some the pasta cooking water. Throw the cooked pasta.

- Set up a medium intensity in a major skillet. Acquire the wine and the shrimp. Close the cover and stew for 1-2 minutes, or until the shrimp become pink and misty.

- Simply remove it from the dish. Put some oil in a dish and sauté a few onions until they're delicate. Cook the garlic briefly. Add the spinach, mix, cover, and let it steam for 2 to 3 minutes. You may now set up the shrimp and pasta. Mix fixings together by blending.

107. Asian-inspired baked fish.

Ingredients:

- 1 pound (455 g) canned halibut fillets

- 1/2 cup (120 ml) (120 ml) Teriyaki sauce with less salt, like Dick's (recipe on page 25).

- (2 Tablespoons) (16 g) The seeds of the sesame plant

- 8 grams flour may be divided into 1 tablespoon.

- one gram of white pepper (half a teaspoon)

Procedure:

- Eggs and milk ought to be combined as one in a little bowl. Put some pepper on it. Shower a pie dish with nonstick vegetable oil splash, then, at that point, spread portion of the cheddar in the base. Spread the cheddar first, then the onions, then get done with the tomatoes. Sprinkle the veggies with the egg combination.

- Season with the excess cheddar and serve. Put it in the broiler and set the clock for 10 minutes. Prepare for 15-20 minutes, or until filling is puffed and brilliant brown, at a decreased intensity of 350°F (180°C or gas mark 4). Serve hot.

- Put filets in a solitary layer on a baking sheet that has been showered with nonstick vegetable oil splash. Cover the highest point of each filet with a little covering of nonstick vegetable oil shower.

- Ten to fifteen minutes, or until fish pieces promptly when punctured with a fork and it is brilliant brown.

108. Fried Fish with a Thai Twist

This Asian fish stew has a wonderful array of flavors and is sure to become a household staple.

Ingredients:

- Catfish fillets weighing 2 pounds (905 g) and sliced into 5-centimeter (2-inch) pieces

- Lemon juice, 1/4 cup (60 ml)

- Sprinkling of red pepper flakes, about a quarter teaspoon's worth (0.3 g)

- 1/2 teaspoon (15 ml) The health benefits of sesame oil

- 1 cup (160 g) (160 g) thinly sliced onion

- **Ingredients:** 1 cup (100 grams) sliced celery; 1 cup (70 grams) shredded bok choy

- Ginger powder, one teaspoon's worth (1.8 g)

- 3 grams of garlic, minced

- 1/2 teaspoon (6.3 g) the spice curry

- 8 cups (1.9 L) (1.9 L) broth made with minimal levels of salt from chicken

- 2 cups (330 g) (330 g) The rice was already cooked.

Procedure:

- Join the catfish with the lime juice and the red pepper drops, and afterward set the combination to the side. In a huge skillet or Dutch broiler, warm the sesame oil. For 1 moment, sauté the onion, celery, bok choy, ginger, and garlic. Use curry powder as a flavoring. Turn the intensity down and cook the onion until it's delicate.

- Place the chicken stock in a pot and intensity to a bubble. Add the catfish combination, and stew for three minutes, or until the fish is cooked. Serve by spooning soup over rice in individual dishes.

109. Salad with Tuna and Pasta

When the weather is hot and you don't feel like cooking, this salad may serve as your main course.

Weighing in at a mere 8 ounces (225 g) Spaghetti made with 100% whole wheat

Ingredients:

- 1/2 pound (225 g) green pods of a pea plant

- There is just enough tuna for one can.

- Size: 6 oz (170 g) Hearts of artichoke

- a half a cup of sliced green olives (around 50 grams)

- 35 grams (1/2 pound) of freshly sliced mushrooms

- 1/2 cup (120 ml) (120 ml) Dressing, Italian

- 1/3 of a teaspoon of lemon pepper

- Grated Parmesan cheese, about a quarter cup (25 g)

Procedure:

Pasta should be cooked to package guidelines, then drained and allowed to cool. Pea pods need just a minute in boiling water before they are ready to be removed and set aside to cool. Gather the empty pods and shells in a container. Tuna, after being rinsed, may be added to a dish of pea pods. Include mushrooms, olives, artichoke hearts, and artichoke juice. Toss with spaghetti and dress with the dressing. Toss in some ground lemon pepper and stir to combine. Put some Parmesan on top.

110. Salad with Tuna, White Beans, and Pasta

One serving of this delicious main course salad provides about half of the recommended daily fiber intake.

Ingredients:

- Vegetables

- Artichoke hearts, one can

- 6 ounces of green beans (170 grams), blanched and drained

- beets, half a pound (225 g), cooked or canned, drained, and sliced

- Tomatoes, cut into wedges (1 1/2 cups/270 g)

- Pasta Mixture

- 225 grams (1/2 pound) of cooked, drained, and washed whole wheat pasta

- 2 cups (200 grams) of cooked, drained white beans

- 1 drained can of tuna

- Vinaigrette

- 60 ml (1/4 cup) of olive oil

- 1/2 cup (120 ml) (120 ml) Lemon juice that has just been squeezed from a lemon

- Minced garlic (one half of a clove)

- 1/2 fresh basil leaf

Procedure:

Mix the vinaigrette ingredients together using a whisk. Marinate the veggies for at least an hour in half of the vinaigrette mixture. Combine the pasta, beans, and tuna in a single bowl once they have been drained. Combine the remaining vinaigrette with the vegetable-pasta combination just before serving.

111. Pasta with Shrimp and Spinach

Flavor is subtle, but you can't go wrong with the health benefits and deliciousness of shrimp and spinach.

Ingredients:

- Whole wheat pasta, 6 ounces

- 1 lb. peeled shrimp

- Two-thirds of a cup of white wine, dry

- Approximately 2 teaspoons of olive oil

- 1 cup of sliced onion

- a minced clove of garlic equaling one teaspoon

- One kilogram of fresh spinach

Procedure:

- It is prescribed to get ready pasta as per bundle rules, barring the utilization of salt. Put away some the pasta cooking water. Throw the cooked pasta. Set up a medium intensity in a major skillet. Get the wine and the shrimp. Close the top and stew for 1-2 minutes, or until the shrimp become pink and obscure.

- Simply remove it from the container. Put some oil in a container and sauté a few onions until they're delicate. Cook the garlic briefly. Add the spinach, mix, cover, and let it steam for 2 to 3 minutes. You may now set up the shrimp and pasta. Mix fixings together by blending.

112. Gravy shrimp

Combination of Shrimp and Scallops Classic seafood paella cooked in a healthy way.

Ingredients:

- Peppers: 1 cup Onion: 1/2 cup Red Bell Peppers: 1 cup

- 1 tablespoon of finely chopped garlic

- 1-half of a teaspoon of turmeric

- A pinch of paprika

- Three and a quarter cups' worth of water

- 1 1/2 cups of uncooked long-grain rice

- 1 pound peeled shrimp 1 cup chopped artichoke hearts

- 12 pound of scallops

- Peas, thawed, 1/2 cup

Procedure:

- Eggs and milk ought to be combined as one in a little bowl. Put some pepper on it. Shower a pie dish with nonstick vegetable oil splash, then, at that point, spread portion of the cheddar in the base. Spread the cheddar first, then the onions, then get done with the tomatoes. Sprinkle the veggies with the egg combination.

- Season with the excess cheddar and serve. Put it in the broiler and set the clock for 10 minutes. Prepare for 15-20 minutes, or until filling is puffed and brilliant brown, at a decreased intensity of 350°F (180°C or gas mark 4). Serve hot.

Chapter 8

Main Dishes: Poultry/Chicken

113. Chicken with a Fruity Honey Mustard Sauce

Um, what more can I say? I was attempting to come up with something novel, when this idea occurred to me. It was created from scratch and is unique. The usual variety should work as well, but I chose tropical fruit cocktail.

Ingredients:

- Six chicken breasts without the bones.
- Fruit cocktail in juice, enough for 1 cup (240 g)
- 1.5 teaspoons (30 ml) acetic acid from red wine
- Two Tablespoons (or 30 ml) of Honey
- Honey mustard, 2 teaspoons (about 30 ml)

Procedure:

- Prepare oven by setting temperature to 180 degrees Celsius (gas mark 4) or 350 degrees Fahrenheit. Put the chicken breasts in a roasting pan. Put the fruit cocktail, vinegar, honey, and mustard in a blender and puree until smooth. To use, just pour over chicken. Put it in the oven and bake for 50 to 60 minutes.

114. Chicken with a Maple Glaze

These grilled chicken breasts are delicious with their maple-mustard glaze.

Ingredients:

- Three-quarters of a cup's worth of maple syrup
- 1/4 cup of Dijon mustard
- 2-tablespoons of minced chives
- 4 chicken breasts, skinned and boneless
- Use a salt-free seasoning mix, such as Mrs. Dash, and add it to the dish at the rate of one
- One-fourth of a teaspoon of pepper

Procedure:

- The grill should be preheated to medium. Combine the syrup, mustard, and chives. Add spice mix and pepper to the chicken. Cook on the grill for 15–20 minutes, basting with sauce every few minutes, or until the meat is no longer pink in the middle. Bring the rest of the sauce to a boil and let it cook for a minute. Prepare to accompany chicken.

115. Snow Peas with Chicken

This has an Asian vibe thanks to the stir-frying and ingredients, but it doesn't employ the customary Asian flavors. It's delicious over rice and probably tastes great with pasta, too.

Ingredients:

- 2 teaspoons (15 g) nonfat dry milk
- Dried parsley, one tablespoon (0.4 grams)
- Paprika, 1 Tablespoon (7 g)
- Onion powder, one teaspoon's worth (3 g)
- **Ingredients:** Garlic powder, about a quarter teaspoon's worth (0.8 g)
- Season poultry with half a teaspoon (0.4 g) of seasoning

Procedure:

- In a wok, warm up 1 tablespoon (15 ml) of the oil. Cover half of the chicken with egg, then roll in cornstarch. Cook in a sautéed food for around four to five minutes, or until delicate.
- Take out the chicken that has been cooked, and afterward do likewise with the remainder of the chicken. Take the chicken out and place the leftover oil in the wok. To cook the onion in a pan-fried food, hold on until it mellows fairly.
- Pan sear the green pepper and snow peas for 4 minutes, or until fresh delicate. Throw the veggies in the honey to cover them. Toss in the chicken and throw until uniformly covered and cooked. Speck the top with almonds.

116. Cooking a Polynesian-style chicken

The citrus fruit chunks in the sauce give this dish a unique twist on traditional sweet-and-sour chicken.

Ingredients:

- Two chicken breasts, each cut in half
- Thighs from 4 chickens
- One grapefruit, three oranges
- 1/2 cup (120 ml) (120 ml) Corn syrup, light
- Mustard, one fourth cup (60 ml)
- Apple cider vinegar, 1/4 cup (60 ml)
- A Spicy Touch with Just a Touch of Tabasco
- ginger, 1/8 teaspoon
- Add 2 tsp. of cornstarch to the mix.
- The equivalent of one tablespoon (15 ml) of water
- 9.2 grams (255 g) pineapple chunks
- Toasted almonds, slivered, 1/3 cup (36 g)

Procedure:

• Put chicken in a small baking dish, skin side down. Cut grapefruit in half while holding it over a dish to collect the juice. Obtain a juice meter. Grapefruit juice is diluted with orange juice to form 1/2 cup (120 ml). Mix together the corn syrup, mustard, vinegar, Tabasco, ginger, and fruit juices in a saucepan. Bring the cornstarch and water mixture to a boil and add it to the pot.

• Bring to a boil and keep stirring for 5 minutes. Use this sauce to brush across chicken. Turn once and baste with sauce while baking for 1 hour at 350 degrees Fahrenheit (180 degrees Celsius, gas mark 4).

• To the leftover sauce, add crushed pineapple, orange, and grapefruit slices, as well as almonds. Warm; drizzle over chicken during the last 5 minutes of baking.

117. Lemon Roasted Chicken with Rosemary

I now prefer using this method whenever I grill chicken. Using this method ensures that the meat does not dry out during cooking and that the outside does not burn. In addition, there is generally enough for sandwiches or salads the following day. If you don't eat the skin, a whole chicken may be a lean source of protein with very little saturated fat.

Ingredients:

• 3–4 pound (1–2) entire chicken (1.4 to 1.8 kg)
• 1/2 a cup of lemon juice (120 ml)
• a pinch of dried rosemary, around 1.2 grams

Procedure:

• Cut the chicken in half lengthwise, through the breastbone and the spine. Combine with lemon juice and fresh rosemary in a resealable plastic bag. Marinate, rotating occasionally, for at least two hours. Get the grill ready by heating one side to high temperature and the other side to low. For approximately an hour, rotating often, cook on low heat. Throw away the peel.

118. Chopped Chicken

Any leftover smoked or barbecued chicken may be put to good use here. If you serve it with the Onion Rolls from Chapter 21 and some coleslaw, you won't even miss the pricey sandwiches at your favorite barbecue restaurant.

Ingredients:

• 16 grams (225 g) The Tomato Sauce with No Salt Added
• Vinegar, about one-fourth cup (60 ml)
• The equivalent of one-fourth cup (60 ml) of molasses
• Powdered onion, equivalent to half a teaspoon (1.5 g)
• Chili powder, equivalent to about a half teaspoon (1.3 g)
• Dry Mustard, 1/2 Teaspoon (1.5 g)

- one-fourth of a teaspoon (0.5 g) hot pepper flakes
- Ingredients Garlic powder, about a quarter teaspoon's worth (0.8 g)
- 1 pound (450 g) smoked chicken, shredded 2 cups

Procedure:

- In a bowl, combine the first eight ingredients (through garlic powder). Add the chicken and mix well, or serve the chicken on top of the rolls with the sauce.

119. The Chicken of Morocco

This chicken meal, inspired by the cuisine of North Africa, has sweet spices that contrast with salty olives and tangy tomatoes.

Ingredients:

- A spoonful of olive oil
- 4 chicken breasts, skinned and boneless
- It weighs 14 ounces. Tomatoes with no additional salt
- one-fourth cup of olives, preferably ripe
- two cups of sliced zucchini
- 1 cup chopped red bell peppers
- 1 Reduced to a half teaspoon, cumin
- a half a teaspoon of cinnamon
- 1-milliliter portion of grated lemon peel

Procedure:

- In a big, nonstick pan, heat the oil over medium heat. Add the chicken and cook for 5 minutes, stirring occasionally, until golden brown. Before serving the chicken, combine the sauce ingredients. Simmer, covered, for 20 minutes, or until the chicken is no longer pink in the middle.

120. Slow-Cooker Chicken Curry

My tongue really like a good curry dish. In a slow cooker, they release a wonderful scent upon completion, making them a pleasant homecoming supper. Multiple curry-typical spices are called for here.

Ingredients:

- Five medium potatoes, diced
- 1 cup peppers, green, roughly chopped
- 1 cup onion, roughly chopped
- 1 pound 2 cups of diced boneless chicken breasts (480 g) canned tomatoes without salt
- a heaping spoonful of ground coriander
- One and a half teaspoons of paprika

- The equivalent of one tablespoon of ginger
- Pepper flakes equal to one-fourth of a teaspoon
- A Half Measure of Turmeric
- Cinnamon, Quarter Teaspoonful
- about equivalent to one-eighth of a teaspoon of cloves
- 1 cup (235 ml) (235 ml) chicken stock without salt
- 2.5 teaspoons (28 ml) chilled liquid
- Four Tablespoons (32 g) cornstarch

Procedure:

- Fill your slow cooker with potatoes, peppers, and onions. Arrange chicken on top. Combine the chicken broth, seasonings, and diced tomatoes. Serve on chicken. To prepare food, set the slow cooker to cook for 8-10 hours, or the high setting for 4-6 hours.
- Take out the meat and the veggies. Maximize the temperature. To make cornstarch, combine it with water. Put into the oven or the stove.
- Incorporate some thickening agents and continue cooking for 15–20 minutes, until sauce reaches desired consistency. Combine the meat and veggies with the sauce.

121. Curry with Chicken and Chickpeas

This is packed with protein thanks to the low-fat chicken and chickpeas, while other veggies offer further nutrients. It's a great way to cut down on carbs without resorting to rice or another starchy staple.

Ingredients:

- 1 cup of nonfat plain yogurt
- Curry powder, 3 tablespoons
- Turmeric, 3 Tablespoons
- a single spoonful of canola oil
- Chicken breasts (boneless, skinless, 12 oz.)
- Lemon juice, 1 tablespoon
- 1 tablespoon of chopped fresh coriander 1/2 teaspoon of minced garlic
- A half cup of chopped onion and green pepper
- Chickpeas, one cupful, cooked

Procedure:

- Canola oil should be heated in a large saucepan before adding the onion, coriander, green peppers, garlic, and chick peas. Use a low heat while frying. Curry and turmeric should be added to the onion mixture. If you feel like you need more liquid, just add more water. Taking out of the oven.

- Fry chicken until it reaches an internal temperature of 165. Put some lemon juice on top and sprinkle. After adding the onion and curry powder, the chicken should simmer for around 20 minutes. After stirring in the yogurt, you can turn off the heat.

122. Baked Chicken and Zucchini

Taking cues from the self-crusting Bisquick impossible pies, this is a simple and delicious one-dish supper.

Ingredients:

- Cooked chicken breast 1 cup (113 g)
- Cubed zucchini 1 cup (180 g)
- In a bowl, whisk together 2 eggs.
- Weight: 225 grams (1 cup) fat-free cottage cheese
- 1 pound (455 g) sliced boneless chicken breast
- 6 ounces Low-sodium tomato paste
- 1 teaspoon (4 g) sugar
- Dried oregano, one teaspoon (1 g)
- 2 eggs
- Exactly one-fourth of a teaspoon (0.5 g) seasoning pepper with black pepper

Procedure:

- Splash a 9-inch (23-cm) pie skillet with nonstick vegetable oil shower and spot in a preheated 400°F (200°C, or gas mark 6) stove. Join the cooked chicken, zucchini, tomato, onion, and cheddar, and spread it out in a pie dish. Mix or whisk the excess fixings together until totally smooth. Pour over chicken blend and spread equitably. Put in the broiler and heat for 35 minutes, or until a blade embedded in the center tells the truth.

- Hold off on the cutting for 5 minutes.

123. Baking a Chicken and Sausage Pie

An authentic rural cuisine, this pie has a cornmeal crust and is stuffed with chicken and sausage.

Ingredients:

- Two potatoes, sliced into 1-centimeter (1/2-inch) cubes
- Breakfast sausage, around 1/2 pound (225 g)
- 1/2 cup cubed carrot
- 2.5 teaspoons (16 g) flour
- In a bowl, whisk together 2 eggs.
- Weight: 225 grams (1 cup) fat-free cottage cheese
- 1 pound (455 g) sliced boneless chicken breast

- 6 ounces Low-sodium tomato paste
- 1 teaspoon (4 g) sugar
- Dried oregano, one teaspoon (1 g)
- A single teaspoon of chicken seasoning
- Crusted in Cornmeal
- Unsalted Butter, 1/4 Cup (55 g)
- 2.5 teaspoons (28 ml) chilled liquid

Procedure:

- Plan potatoes by bubbling them until they are fork-delicate. Channel. Frankfurter ought to be disintegrated and set in a major, profound dish. Incorporate the chicken. Put the oven on medium intensity.

- For roughly 5 minutes, or until the celery and carrot are cooked, add the onion, garlic powder, and a spot of salt. Mix the flour, wine, and stock together.

- Put into pot and intensity till bubbling. Lessen intensity and stew until thick and gurgling, then season with thyme and poultry zest and mix in potatoes.

124. Mousaka made with zucchini

Instead of the more traditional lamb and eggplant, this Greek recipe uses minced turkey and zucchini.

Ingredients:

- 675 grams (six cups) of sliced zucchini

- Turkey ground, about a half pound (225 grams)

- 1 cup of chopped onion (about 160 grams) 2 tablespoons of minced garlic (about 6 grams)

- 12 teaspoon (1.2 g) cinnamon

- In a bowl, whisk together 2 eggs.

- Weight: 225 grams (1 cup) fat-free cottage cheese

- 1 pound (455 g) sliced boneless chicken breast

- 6 ounces Low-sodium tomato paste

- 1 teaspoon (4 g) sugar

- Dried oregano, one teaspoon (1 g)

- In a bowl, whisk together 2 eggs.

- Exactly one-fourth of a teaspoon (0.6 g) nutmeg

Procedure:

• Set broiler temperature to 350F (180C)/gas mark 4. Oil a little baking dish that holds 2 quarts (1.9 liters) of fluid. In a major, nonstick dish, bring 3 cups (705 ml) of water to a bubble. Throw in the zucchini, cover, and bubble for 10 minutes, or until fresh delicate.

• Assume out and position on some paper towels to absorb the abundance water. The container should have been cleaned down. Cook the turkey with the onions and garlic. Ensure the turkey is very much cooked through.

• Cinnamon and oregano might be added to the stock and rice after they have been blended together. Ten minutes covered at a stew, blending two times or threefold. Toss some pureed tomatoes in with the general mish-mash.

• Add the milk gradually while blending. Whisk every now and again for 4-5 minutes until the combination thickens and becomes smooth. Throw the eggs with 33% of the hot sauce, then, at that point, add the egg-sauce blend to the remainder of the sauce and throw. Remove the oven and blend in the nutmeg.

125. Grilled Roaster

On the weekend, you may have a delicious supper and enough of leftovers to utilize throughout the week. Flavor-wise, this one is smokey without being overpowering.

Ingredients:

• 1 big (5-6 lb.) chicken for roasting (2.3 to 2.7 kg)
• Extra-virgin olive oil, 2 teaspoons (30 ml)
• Paprika, one teaspoon's worth (around 2.5 grams)
• 1 tsp. onion powder (3 g)
• 1 gram (about half a teaspoon) of black pepper
• About a half a teaspoon (0.5 g) Thyme, dried
• Garlic powder, equivalent to about a quarter teaspoon (0.8 g)
• The equivalent of one teaspoon (5 ml) of liquid smoke

Procedure:

• The natural division of a chicken into two halves is along the backbone and the breastbone.

• Make a rub out of the remaining ingredients and apply to both sides of the chicken halves. It takes anything from 1 1/2 to 2 hours on the grill over indirect heat, rotating periodically.

• The remaining 15 minutes, while trying to achieve a browning effect, should be spent in a low oven.

126. Breasts of Chicken with a Rotisserie Flavor

In this dish, leaner chicken breasts are used to create a taste similar to takeout rotisserie chicken.

Ingredients:

- One-fourth of a cup (60 ml) of honey
- Paprika, one teaspoon's worth (around 2.5 grams)
- Onion powder, 1 teaspoon (3 grams)
- A half-teaspoonful of black pepper (1 gram)
- Thieves' thyme, dried, 1/2 teaspoon (0.5 g)
- Garlic powder, equivalent to about a quarter teaspoon (0.8 g)
- (4 boneless chicken breasts)

Procedure:

- Prepare a 325F (170C or gas mark 3) oven. Prepare a seasoning blend using honey, paprika, onion powder, black pepper, thyme, and garlic powder. Mix together and use on chicken. Toss every 15 minutes with the pan juices and roast for 45 minutes.

127. Chicken breasts marinated in a grilling sauce

These sliced, grilled chicken breasts are perfect for lunchtime sandwiches. Sliced and added to a salad or mixed into a pasta salad, they're delicious.

Ingredients:

- 60 ml (one-fourth of a cup) of olive oil
- A little bit of red wine, around a quarter cup (60 ml) vinegar
- The equivalent of one-fourth of a teaspoon (0.8 g) of minced garlic
- Onion powder, 1 teaspoon (3 grams)
- 1 and a half teaspoons (1 g) of Italian seasoning
- Thieves' thyme, dried, 1/2 teaspoon (0.5 g)
- Two chicken breasts without the bones.

Procedure:

- Put everything except the chicken in a resealable plastic bag and stir until everything is evenly distributed.
- In order to form two thin fillets, cut each breast in half lengthwise. Marinate the chicken for at least two hours in the fridge, rotating the bag occasionally. After that, seal it.
- Chicken may be grilled over medium heat, turned once, until cooked through.

128. Vegetables and chicken on the grill.

Grilled chicken and veggies marinated with lemon and herbs.

Ingredients:

- a half a teaspoon of basil
- 1/2 teaspoon of dried garlic
- Black pepper, one-fourth teaspoon
- a single gated teaspoon of lemon peel
- 1/4 cup water 1 tbsp. lemon juice
- Approximately 1 Tablespoon of Olive Oil
- Four skinless, boneless chicken breasts
- 1-ounces of sliced eggplant
- 1-inch lengthwise slices of zucchini
- Crosswise cut 1 red bell pepper

Procedure:

- Add the first six ingredients together. Prepare a grilling medium-heat temperature. Use the herb combination as a brushing sauce for poultry and veggies. To prevent the chicken from becoming pink in the middle, grill it for 5-10 minutes each side. Cook veggies on the grill for approximately 5 minutes each side, or until they are crisp tender.

129. Kabobs with Italian-style chicken

These delectable kabobs, which are like pizza on a stick, will be a hit with guests of all ages.

Ingredients:

- 1 lb. of boneless, skinless chicken breast, diced into 1" cubes
- 1 cup of chopped green bell peppers, about one inch long
- 1 cup of sliced red bell peppers (1 inch chunks)
- eight ounces of mushrooms
- A Reduced-Fat (1/4 Cup) Toppings from Italy (recipe in Chapter 2)
- Mix in 1 teaspoon of Italian seasoning
- Grated Parmesan: 14 cup

Procedure:

- Grill should be preheated to medium heat. Meat and produce may be skewered and then grilled. Sprinkling Italian spice and brushing with dressing. Chicken has to be grilled for approximately 10 minutes, or until the middle is no longer pink. Take them off the skewers and top with cheese.

130. A Chicken Dish with Lemon and Thyme

These grilled chicken breasts have a sweet and tart taste because to the combination of honey and lemon.

Ingredients:

- To sweeten: 1/4 cup honey
- Grated lemon peel equal to 1 Tablespoon
- 1/4 cup water 1 tbsp. lemon juice
- Approximately one-half teaspoon of thyme
- Black pepper, one-fourth teaspoon
- Four chicken breasts without the bones and skin

Procedure:

- Bring grill up to medium heat. Add pepper and thyme to honey and lemon juice. After around 15–20 minutes on the grill, the chicken should be well cooked through.
- Apply the sauce with a brush during the final ten minutes of cooking.

131. Fried Chicken Made in the Oven

Healthy alternatives to traditional fried chicken exist. Chicken is a healthy option after you remove the skin and "fry" it in the oven. And it has a pleasant flavor to boot!

Ingredients:

- 55 grams (a quarter cup) of unsalted butter, melted
- a half gram (0.14) of black pepper
- Remove skin and bone from 3 pounds (1.4 kg) of chicken and chop into bite-sized pieces.
- Breadcrumbs made from corn flakes, 1 cup (56 g)

Procedure:

- The recommended oven temperature is 350 degrees Fahrenheit (180 degrees Celsius, or gas mark 4). The butter and pepper should be mixed together. Coat the chicken with the butter-and-herbs mixture, then roll it in corn flakes. Put in a pan without greasing it and bake for 1 hour.

132. Chicken with a Potato Coating and Oven Fry

In my opinion, this is the best chicken to bake in the oven.

Ingredients:

* 1 egg
* The equivalent of 2 teaspoons (30 ml) of water
* 1/4 cup (25 g) (25 g) 3 pounds (1.4 kilograms) of chicken, boned and skinned
* 1 cup (60 g) (60 g) A packet of instant mashed potatoes

Procedure:

* Have prepared a stove preheated to 375 degrees Fahrenheit (190 degrees Celsius, or gas mark 5). In a blending bowl, whisk together the egg, water, and cheddar.
* Roll chicken in potato flakes after dipping it in an egg and milk combination. Set in a pan for baking that has not been oiled. Bake for one hour after placing in oven.

133. Baked Chicken Nuggets

Chicken nuggets are far healthier if baked rather than fried. They taste exactly the same but have much fewer negative health effects.

Ingredients:

* 1/2 cup Corn flakes, crushed
* 2 teaspoons (15 g) nonfat dry milk
* Dried parsley, one tablespoon (0.4 grams)
* Paprika, 1 Tablespoon (7 g)
* Onion powder, one teaspoon's worth (3 g)
* Garlic powder, about a quarter teaspoon's worth (0.8 g)
* Season poultry with half a teaspoon (0.4 g) of seasoning
* Boneless chicken breasts weighing 1 pound (455 g)
* Single egg, beaten

Procedure:

* Plan broiler by setting temperature to 180 degrees Celsius (gas mark 4) or 350 degrees Fahrenheit. In a resealable plastic pack, join squashed corn drops with the accompanying six fixings (through poultry preparing).
* The chicken should be dipped in egg before being placed in the bag. If you want a uniform coating, give it a good shake. Put on a baking sheet sprayed with vegetable oil spray that won't make the food cling. Cook chicken and crisp up the coating in the oven for 20 minutes.

134. Spaghetti and Chicken Bake

My daughter's culinary tenet is basically this: when in doubt about what to prepare for supper, go Italian. I'm satisfied with that solution!

Ingredients:

- pasta, 8 ounces (or 225 grams)

- In a bowl, whisk together 2 eggs.

- Weight: 225 grams (1 cup) fat-free cottage cheese

- 1 pound (455 g) sliced boneless chicken breast

- 6 ounces Low-sodium tomato paste

- 1 teaspoon (4 g) sugar

- Dried oregano, one teaspoon (1 g)

- 1/2 teaspoon (1.5 g) garlic powder

- mozzarella cheese, shredded; 1/2 cup (60 g)

Procedure:

- Set oven temperature to 350F. Prepare spaghetti as directed on the box. Drain. incorporate eggs Create a "crust" with the dough and place it into a prepared 10-inch (25-cm) pie pan.

- Cottage cheese goes well on top. Cook chicken, onion, and green bell pepper in a large pan until chicken is cooked through and onion and pepper are soft. Incorporate the other ingredients, except from the mozzarella, and warm through. Blend and use as a sauce for pasta and cottage cheese.

- Put the dish in the oven and set the timer for 20 minutes. Top with mozzarella cheese approximately 5 minutes before the conclusion of baking.

135. Tossed Pasta with Chicken and Veggies

Some fresh veggies may be used in this dish. Our options were limited by the materials at hand, but you may adapt them to your own needs. It's great as a warm-weather one-dish supper with some handmade bread on the side.

Ingredients:

- The weight of 8 ounces (225 g) pasta, such as linguine or spaghetti
- Two Tablespoons' Worth (or 30 ml) of Olive Oil
- Zucchini, sliced into thin strips, 1 cup (113 grams)
- Thinly sliced mushrooms (around 35 grams) equaling 1/2 cup (1 (0.3 g) Basil, Dried
- Garlic, minced, 1/2 teaspoon (1.5 g)

- The equivalent of 1 cup (235 ml) of skim milk
- 2 cups (220 grams) of cooked, diced chicken breast
- 2 tablespoons (10 g) grated Parmesan cheese 1 cup (180 g) sliced roma tomatoes
- 0.3 grams or 1/8 teaspoon black pepper

Procedure:

- Linguine and spaghetti should be prepared as directed on the box. In the meanwhile, get a pan nice and hot and fill it with oil. Flake in some garlic and basil, then throw in some mushrooms and zucchini. Stirring occasionally, cook for 20 to 30 minutes, or until zucchini is just soft. Pasta should be drained and re-added to the pot. Heat through the milk, chicken, and zucchini combination by stirring. Put in some pepper, cheese, and tomatoes. Mix and serve.

136. Tomato, Chicken, and Asparagus Pasta

This delicious and easy main meal is made even better by a light dressing made of Balsamic vinegar and oil.

Ingredients:

- Whole wheat pasta, like rotini, 8 ounces
- 1 pound of boneless, skinless chicken breasts, sliced into 14-inch strips
- 1/4 of a teaspoon of freshly ground black pepper
- 1 cup of sliced asparagus, 1 inch thick
- 1 cup of halved cherry tomatoes
- a half of a teaspoon of minced garlic
- A Half Measure of Basil
- The equivalent of 2 teaspoons of balsamic vinegar
- 2 teaspoons butter

Procedure:

- Follow the instructions on the box for cooking the pasta, but don't add any salt. In a nonstick skillet, bring the fire up to medium heat. Throw in some chicken and asparagus, and cook until the chicken is no longer pink, approximately 5 minutes. Once the tomatoes and garlic are added, continue cooking for another minute. Put the pasta and the rest of the ingredients in a bowl and mix them together when you've taken them from the heat.

A 30 DAYS MEAL PLAN

1ST 10 DAYS	2ND 10 DAYS	3RD 10 DAYS
DAY-1	**DAY-11**	**DAY-21**
Breakfast: Stuffed Mushrooms **Lunch:** Salmon Patties **Dinner:** Tomato, Chicken, and Asparagus Pasta	**Breakfast:** Turkey Breakfast Sausage **Lunch:** Bowl of Chicken Barley Chowder **Dinner:** Tossed Pasta with Chicken and Veggies	**Breakfast:** Cookies for Breaking the Fast **Lunch:** Sashimi-Style Poached Salmon **Dinner:** Spaghetti and Chicken Bake.
DAY-2	**DAY-12**	**DAY-22**
Breakfast: Breakfast in the Snow Casserole **Lunch:** Portobello Mushrooms on the Grill **Dinner:** Baked Chicken Nuggets	**Breakfast:** Vegetable Omelet **Lunch:** Tomato-Chicken Soup **Dinner:** Chicken with a Potato Coating and Oven Fry	**Breakfast:** Baked Spinach **Lunch:** Salad with Tuna and Pasta **Dinner:** Chicken with a Fruity Honey Mustard Sauce
DAY-3	**DAY-13**	**DAY-23**
Breakfast: Skillet for Breakfast **Lunch:** Soup with Italian Chicken **Dinner:** Mousaka made with zucchini	**Breakfast:** Baked Spinach **Lunch:** Salad with Tuna and Pasta **Dinner:** Chicken with a Fruity Honey Mustard Sauce	**Breakfast:** Omelet with cinnamon and apples **Lunch:** Kabobs with Italian-style chicken **Dinner:** Mediterranean Tilapia
DAY-4	**DAY-14**	**DAY-24**
Breakfast: Cookies for Breaking the Fast **Lunch:** Sashimi-Style Poached Salmon **Dinner:** Spaghetti and Chicken Bake.	**Breakfast:** Crepes made with cornmeal **Lunch:** Curry with Chicken and Chickpeas **Dinner:** A Scallop-Topped Linguine Dish	**Breakfast:** Vegetable Omelet **Lunch:** Tomato-Chicken Soup **Dinner:** Chicken with a Potato Coating and Oven Fry

DAY-5	DAY-15	DAY-25
Breakfast: Baked Spinach **Lunch:** Salad with Tuna and Pasta **Dinner:** Chicken with a Fruity Honey Mustard Sauce	**Breakfast:** Skillet for Breakfast **Lunch:** Soup with Italian Chicken **Dinner:** Mousaka made with zucchini	**Breakfast:** Breakfast in the Snow Casserole **Lunch:** Portobello Mushrooms on the Grill **Dinner:** Baked Chicken Nuggets
DAY-6	**DAY-16**	**DAY-26**
Breakfast: Turkey Breakfast Sausage **Lunch:** Bowl of Chicken Barley Chowder **Dinner:** Tossed Pasta with Chicken and Veggies	**Breakfast:** Tomatoes with Stuffing **Lunch:** A Chicken Dish with Lemon and Thyme **Dinner:** Pan-Fried Catfish with Pecans	**Breakfast:** Crepes made with cornmeal **Lunch:** Curry with Chicken and Chickpeas **Dinner:** A Scallop-Topped Linguine Dish
DAY-7	**DAY-17**	**DAY-27**
Breakfast: Vegetable Omelet **Lunch:** Tomato-Chicken Soup **Dinner:** Chicken with a Potato Coating and Oven Fry	**Breakfast:** Omelet with cinnamon and apples **Lunch:** Kabobs with Italian-style chicken **Dinner:** Mediterranean Tilapia	**Breakfast:** Stuffed Mushrooms **Lunch:** Salmon Patties **Dinner:** Tomato, Chicken, and Asparagus Pasta
DAY-8	**DAY-18**	**DAY-28**
Breakfast: Tomatoes with Stuffing **Lunch:** A Chicken Dish with Lemon and Thyme **Dinner:** Pan-Fried Catfish with Pecans	**Breakfast:** Cookies for Breaking the Fast **Lunch:** Sashimi-Style Poached Salmon **Dinner:** Spaghetti and Chicken Bake.	**Breakfast:** Skillet for Breakfast **Lunch:** Soup with Italian Chicken **Dinner:** Mousaka made with zucchini

DAY-9	DAY-19	DAY-29
Breakfast: Crepes made with cornmeal **Lunch:** Curry with Chicken and Chickpeas **Dinner:** A Scallop-Topped Linguine Dish	**Breakfast:** Breakfast in the Snow Casserole **Lunch:** Portobello Mushrooms on the Grill **Dinner:** Baked Chicken Nuggets	**Breakfast:** Tomatoes with Stuffing **Lunch:** A Chicken Dish with Lemon and Thyme **Dinner:** Pan-Fried Catfish with Pecans
DAY-10	**DAY-20**	**DAY-30**
Breakfast: Omelet with cinnamon and apples **Lunch:** Kabobs with Italian-style chicken **Dinner:** Mediterranean Tilapia	**Breakfast:** Stuffed Mushrooms **Lunch:** Salmon Patties **Dinner:** Tomato, Chicken, and Asparagus Pasta	**Breakfast:** Turkey Breakfast Sausage **Lunch:** Bowl of Chicken Barley Chowder **Dinner:** Tossed Pasta with Chicken and Veggies

Conclusion

Controlling diabetes is not a simple task. However, there is no life-threatening sickness. However, don't allow the adjustments in your diet that you need to make in order to alleviate your symptoms to have a negative impact on the quality of your life. At the very least, try not to make the symptoms that are currently present much worse. You are free to consume as much food as you could ever want without putting your health in jeopardy. You need to have the ability to make decisions about the ingredients and recipes that you use. You may begin by following the seven-day food plan that is included in this cookbook and then go from there.

When you start reading through the pages of this recipe book, you will come to the realization that it is possible to have meals that are both nutritious and enjoyable, even if you have diabetes. You are even allowed to indulge in a few sweet treats in between. As long as you are aware of what constitutes diabetic-friendly cuisine, all you need to do is learn how to regulate your portion sizes. It may be challenging to control diabetes, but if you make major adjustments to your lifestyle, you will be able to manage it. It is in your best interest to seek the advice of a qualified medical practitioner who can show you the path to a healthy you. Additionally, keep in mind that you do not have to endure the monotony of eating boring meals every mealtime. You may maintain their interest by preparing foods that are both wholesome and healthy, such as the ones that we have prepared for you in this issue.

Made in the USA
Middletown, DE
05 December 2024